Research in Communication Sciences and Disorders

Methods—Applications—Evaluation

Timothy Meline

University of Texas, Pan American

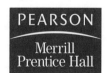

PEARSON

Merrill
Prentice Hall

Upper Saddle River, New Jersey
Columbus, Ohio

Library of Congress Cataloging in Publication Data

Meline, Timothy J.
 Evaluating research for communication disorders : case / Timothy Meline.
     p. cm.
 Includes bibliographical references and index.
 ISBN 0-13-183774-5 (alk. paper)
 1. Communicative disorders--Research--Methodology.   2. Research--Methodology.   I. Title.
 RC337.M45 2006
 616.85'5'072--dc22

                                                    2005014012

Vice President and Executive Publisher: Jeffery W. Johnston
Senior Editor: Allyson P. Sharp
Editorial Assistant: Kathleen S. Burk
Production Editor: Sheryl Langner
Production Coordination: Mike Remillard, Pine Tree Composition, Inc.
Design Coordinator: Diane C. Lorenzo
Cover Design: Jeff Vanik
Cover Image: Corbis
Production Manager: Laura Messerly
Director of Marketing: Ann Castel Davis
Marketing Manager: Autumn Purdy
Marketing Coordinator: Brian Mounts

This book was set in Berkeley by Pine Tree Composition, Inc. It was printed and bound by R. R. Donnelley & Sons Company. The cover was printed by R. R. Donnelley & Sons Company.

Pearson Education Ltd.
Pearson Education Singapore Pte. Ltd.
Pearson Education Canada, Ltd.
Pearson Education–Japan

Pearson Education Australia Pty. Limited
Pearson Education North Asia Ltd.
Pearson Educación de Mexico, S.A. de C.V.
Pearson Education Malaysia Pte. Ltd.

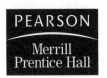

10 9 8 7 6 5 4 3 2
0-13-183774-5

To
Jessie, Noelle, Sebastian, and Willow

PREFACE

The research enterprise is exciting and challenging—exciting in its discovery of new ideas and challenging in its rigorous methods. The importance of research for speech-language pathologists and audiologists is evident in the search for knowledge and the many contributions of research to clinical practice. In notable treatises on research, Wambaugh and Bain (2002) examined the "great need and potential for the application of research to clinical practice," and Brobeck and Lubinsky (2003) promoted the use of single-subject research in clinical practice. Teachers of research methods regularly communicate their enthusiasm for research to students, but students benefit most from hands-on experience. Most programs in communication sciences and disorders recognize the importance of the research experience for undergraduates (Mueller & Lisko, 2003) as well as for graduate students. As Mueller and Lisko advised: "Students who design, fully execute, and disseminate a research project learn to appreciate the excitement of discovery and the reward of scholarship" (p. 124). Williams and Fagelson (2003) recounted their revision of the traditional research pedagogy as a "cooperative learning community"—with journal clubs and collaborative research projects to spur learning. Many programs have adopted similar models in their curriculum, and many students have subsequently presented their research projects in state and national forums. The more research experiences are invested in the undergraduate and graduate curricula, the more students will appreciate the value of research for clinical practice. Students may also recognize research as a legitimate choice for their careers.

To these ends, this text begins with the science that underpins research methods—and ends with an exposition on writing for presentation and publication. The intervening chapters extol many important and diverse issues in research, including ethics, group designs, single-case designs, qualitative designs, survey methods, quantitative methods, research synthesis, evaluating research for practice (evidence-based practice), and more.

The chapters include *Technology Notes* to encourage students to appreciate and explore the modern technology available for research in communication disorders. Throughout the chapters, *Thought Questions* follow case examples to encourage active learning. Nonetheless, there is much unsaid. Students will benefit from an elementary course in research methods, statistics, or quantitative methods in the undergraduate curriculum. As supplements, there are many excellent tutorials in communication disorders journals that address specialized and advanced topics in research. There are also Internet resources available as supplements—and selected Websites are referenced throughout the book.

The twelve chapters are comprehensive in scope, though individual chapters survey their respective topics. For an in-depth treatment of any one topic, students should seek textbooks that are dedicated to that topic. Chapter 1 presents the foundation for scientific inquiry with discussions of the basic principles of science, various types of research, variables and operational definitions, and validity issues.

Chapter 2 is an introduction to ethics in research. It provides a history of ethics, presents professional codes of ethics, discusses the impact of various issues in ethics, and forms the relationship between evidence-based practice and ethics.

Chapter 3 addresses the basic principles underlying scientific observations, including levels of measurement and data collection issues. In addition, it introduces the use of descriptive statistics and visual presentation (statistical graphics) in communication disorders research.

Chapter 4 introduces the foundation for using group research designs in communication disorders, including sampling methods and subject selection procedures. In addition, it introduces complex research designs and their uses in communication disorders research.

Chapter 5 is a survey of qualitative research and its applications to communication disorders research. It includes an orientation to qualitative research and a discussion of basic qualitative research designs with examples. In addition, Chapter 5 discusses credibility and transferability issues related to qualitative research outcomes and the combining of qualitative with quantitative approaches to research in communication disorders.

Chapter 6 is a survey of single-case designs and their applications in communication disorders research. It presents the basic A-B-A, multiple-baseline, changing-criterion, and simultaneous-treatment designs with exemplars.

Chapter 7 presents alternative research designs, including case studies and historical, correlational, developmental, and survey types of research designs. In addition, replication designs, including conceptual, systematic, and direct types, are discussed.

Chapter 8 introduces the topic of hypothesis testing in communication sciences and disorders. It outlines six steps in the hypothesis testing process and introduces the concepts of the normal distribution, standard normal distribution, distribution of test statistics, and the Central Limit Theorem.

Chapter 9 is a review of quantitative analysis methods in communication disorders research, including tests for differences between two groups, simple analysis of variance, complex analysis of variance, and tests for analyzing categorical data.

Chapter 10 introduces the notion of synthesizing research in communication sciences and disorders. It includes a review of a "Model for Clinical-Outcome Research" and presents examples of synthesizing research outcomes by narrative review and quantitative review with step-by-step guidance.

Chapter 11 introduces the topic of evaluating research in communication sciences and disorders for clinical practice. It includes critical questions for evaluation, case examples, and a checklist for critically evaluating research articles.

Chapter 12 introduces the topic of writing for research in communication sciences and disorders, and it includes a review of writing stages, including prewriting/planning, writing/drafting, rewriting/revision, editing, and publication/presentation stages.

Appendix A includes a reprint of the article *Evidence-Based Practice in Schools: Evaluating Research and Reducing Barriers*. It is included as supplemental reading for research issues in evidence-based practice.

Research in Communication Sciences and Disorders presents a cohesive and comprehensive introduction to research for advanced undergraduate students or graduate students in communication sciences and disorders. It was written with the philosophy that no one research design or method is pre-eminent. Each and every method and approach to research has its place—and each one contributes in its unique way. The characteristics that best define quality research are rigorous planning and execution, not the choice of design or methodology.

Acknowledgments

A special appreciation is warranted for the expert reviewers who helped eliminate errors and identified lapses in clarity. Their assistance was invaluable. Thank you to Anne K. Bothe, *University of Georgia;* Stefan A. Frisch, *University of South Florida;* Cheryl D. Gunter, *West Chester University;* Carolyn Wiles Higdon, *University of Mississippi;* Kim McCullough, *University of Central Arkansas;* Kerri Phillips, *Louisiana Tech University;* Steven L. Skelton, *California State University, Fresno;* and Virginia G. Walker, *Florida State University.*

DISCOVER THE MERRILL EDUCATION RESOURCES FOR COMMUNICATION DISORDERS WEBSITE

Technology is a constantly growing and changing aspect of our field that is creating a need for new content and resources. To address this emerging need, Merrill Education has developed an online learning environment for students, teachers, and professors alike to complement our products—the *Merrill Education Resources for Communication Disorders* Website. This content-rich Website provides additional resources specific to this book's topic and will help you—professors, classroom teachers, and students—augment your teaching, learning, and professional development.

Our goal is to build on and enhance what our products already offer. For this reason, the content for our user-friendly Website is organized by topic and provides teachers, professors, and students with a variety of meaningful resources all in one location. With this Website, we bring together the best of what Merrill has to offer: text resources, video clips, Web links, tutorials, and a wide variety of information on topics of interest to general and special educators alike. Rich content, applications, and competencies further enhance the learning process.

The *Merrill Education Resources for Communication Disorders* Website includes:

Resources for the Professor–

- The **Syllabus Manager™**, an online syllabus creation and management tool, enables instructors to create and revise their syllabus with an easy, step-by-step process. Students can access your syllabus and any changes you make during the course of your class from any computer with Internet access. To access this tailored syllabus, students will just need the URL of the Website and the password assigned to the syllabus. By clicking on the date, the student can see a list of activities, assignments, and readings due for that particular class.
- In addition to the **Syllabus Manager™** and its benefits listed above, professors also have access to all of the wonderful resources that students have access to on the site.

Resources for the Student–

- Video clips specific to each topic, with questions to help you evaluate the content and make crucial theory-to-practice connections.
- Thought-provoking critical analysis questions that students can answer and turn in for evaluation or that can serve as basis for class discussions and lectures.
- Access to a wide variety of resources related to classroom strategies and methods, including lesson planning and classroom management.
- Information on all the most current relevant topics related to special and general education, including CEC and Praxis standards, IEPs, portfolios, and professional development.
- Extensive Web resources and overviews on each topic addressed on the Website.
- A message board with discussion starters where students can respond to class discussion topics, post questions and responses, or ask questions about assignments.
- A search feature to help access specific information quickly.

To take advantage of these and other resources, please visit the *Merrill Education Resources for Communication Disorders* Website at:

http://www.prenhall.com/meline

BRIEF CONTENTS

CONTENTS

7   Alternative Designs in Communication Disorders Research   100

Note: Every effort has been made to provide accurate and current Internet information in this book. However, the Internet and information posted on it are constantly changing, so it is inevitable that some of the Internet addresses listed in this textbook will change.

PART I

Foundations of Science and Research in Communication Disorders

1 Scientific Inquiry in Communication Disorders Research

re · search   (rí-sûrch') v. analyze, experiment, explore, inquire, investigate, probe, scrutinize, study.

Scientific inquiry aims to better understand the world and its inhabitants. This goal is achieved by accumulating a body of scientific knowledge. In daily life, information is gathered from many sources—including newspapers, magazines, books, and the internet, as well as from friends, coworkers, newscasters, and experts who share their professional opinions. Information is also gathered from personal experiences with the world and its inhabitants—though personal experiences are mediated by the senses as well as past experiences. In this regard, Borden, Harris, and Raphael (2002) explained: "Our perceptions often match our expectations rather than what was actually said and heard" (p. 151). Borden et al. (2002) referred to this characteristic of human perception as *duality*. In the ordinary world, these *ways of knowing the world* may be acceptable guides for daily living—but science imposes a higher standard of objectivity and reliability than ordinary observations allow. The *scientific method* prescribes a set of rules and principles that guide the search for knowledge.

The Scientific Method

Scientists attempt to describe the world and logically organize the information that is collected into the larger body of knowledge. *Research* is the process whereby scientists attempt to understand the world and its inhabitants. Scientific research is governed by a rigid set of rules that define the scientific method. Three important assumptions are the underpinnings of the scientific method:

1. *Order:* Scientists believe that events occur in regular patterns—not random occurrences.
2. *Determinism:* Scientists believe that the occurrence of an event is determined by prior events.
3. *Discoverability:* Scientists expect to find answers to research questions. However, new questions arise as others are answered. In this way, scientific research is an ongoing and continuous process of discovery.

Scientific Observations

Scientists observe events to explain the relationship between two or more variables. *Variables* are properties that take on different values—as few as two up to an infinite number. The scientific method imposes several conditions on observations. First, observations must be objective. *Objectivity* is the expression of reality without the intrusion of the researchers' personal beliefs, biases, or emotions. Speculation about unobserved events is expressly prohibited. Second, the events and observations of events must be *public*—because science is a social enterprise and the research process should be open to scrutiny by all. Third, observations must be *repeatable*. A research study must be described in enough detail to allow others to replicate its methods and results. The replication process provides for a *confirmation* of results. The need to confirm or refute research results is basic to the scientific approach. Nothing is assumed to be true until it is confirmed by independent investigations.

Cause and Effect

Sometimes researchers in communication disorders observe people and events without inferring causality. For example, some studies are interested in the relationship between two variables such as gender and perceptions of hearing-aid use with no consideration of causality; others may survey opinions about professional issues without inferring

Technology Note

Technology is more than electronic and digital products. Its definition includes the application of science and the materials (or resources) used to achieve scientific objectives. An especially important resource for achieving scientific objectives is the brain power provided by individuals in the discipline of communication disorders. The American Speech-Language-Hearing Association's Research and Scientific Affairs Committee highlighted the need for a strong research base in the professions because of the interdependence of practitioners and researchers. The Committee recommended a reemphasis on research methods in training programs, along with experiences in conducting research (American Speech-Language-Hearing Association, 1994).

causality. Nonetheless, most research in communication disorders is interested in cause-effect relationships at some point in time.

Typically, researchers infer cause from effect by eliminating all other possible causes. The cause-effect relationship is stated as: *If A then B*. There are three conditions for inferring causality: (a) the treatment occurs before the change—not after, (b) the change is observable, and (c) no other variable can account for the change. The third condition is rarely achieved because variables are not easily isolated. Thus, the relationship is stated as: *A implies B*. Researchers use *statistics* to verify implications such as $A \rightarrow B$.

Steps in the Scientific Method

Ideas for research come from a variety of sources. For example, speech-language pathology and audiology practices are excellent sources of ideas for scientific study. Clinical experiences, anecdotal accounts, and case studies may inspire future investigations. Likewise, social, political, and regulatory demands for quality assurance are catalysts for studies of treatment efficacy. On the other hand, research reports, articles, editorials, letters to the editor, and textbooks in communication disorders are rich sources of ideas.

Once the seed of an idea exists or a problem to be solved is identified, it must be expressed in a manageable way. The scientific principle of objectivity requires formality throughout the research process. As a consequence, observations are usually coded so that they can be reliably recorded. In addition, *operational definitions* are written for each variable of interest. An operational definition gives meaning to a variable by specifying the activities necessary for its measurement. There are *five major steps* in the scientific process as follow:

1. *Statement of the problem:* The statement of the problem should be a clear description of the problem along with a rationale for its study. Research questions are usually evident once the problem to be addressed is clear. The research questions should express the goals of the study.
2. *The research hypothesis:* Another step in the research process is the formulation of the research hypothesis. In Friedman's words: "The construction of hypotheses is a creative act of inspiration, intuition, invention; its essence is the vision of something new in familiar material" (1953, p. 43). A hypothesis is a best guess as to the answer to a research question. The research hypothesis should be supported by the existing scientific literature, as well as personal experiences.
3. *The research method:* A third critical step in the research process is to develop a procedure for answering the research questions. The *research method* includes a specification of participants and a detailed plan for observing behaviors and recording data. Observations become data when they are coded in some operational form. A numerical coding is most common because numbers are easily recorded, analyzed, and stored. Numerical coding is the hallmark of quantitative research. On the other hand, qualitative research methods depend on descriptions, categories, and words for data. Whatever the nature of the data (quantitative or qualitative), a research study's success depends on the *validity* and *reliability* of its methods. Validity has to do with the meaningfulness of results; reliability has to do with the ability to replicate results.

4. *The analysis of results:* After collecting and recording the data, researchers analyze it. A typical analysis includes graphs, tables, and statistics. The different kinds of analyses help to accurately interpret results. If the analysis of data is faulty, the research conclusions will be faulty. For this reason, the analysis of data is an especially rigorous and demanding step in the research process. Researchers may seek advice from statisticians and other experts in data analysis because this step in the research process is highly specialized.

5. *Interpretation of results:* The interpretation of results is guided by both the research questions and hypotheses that were originally proposed. The goals for the interpretation of results are: (a) to answer each research question, and (b) to support or refute the hypothesis. Sometimes, new research questions, as well as methodological shortcomings, are revealed when data are analyzed and interpreted. The interpretation of results is typically included in the *conclusion* section at the end of the research report.

Types of Research in Communication Disorders

By convention, research is organized into various divisions—and some are dichotomous. In practice, the boundaries that divide one type of research from another are artificial and often overlap. Nonetheless, these divisions are a basis for understanding the complexities of research designs.

Basic and Applied Research

The simplest way to distinguish between basic and applied types of research is to examine the purpose for conducting a research study. If the sole purpose is to contribute new scientific knowledge with no intention of solving a social or clinical problem or any other practical application, the research is best described as *basic research*. On the other hand, if the purpose is clearly to solve a social problem, clinical problem, or other practical application, the research is best described as *applied research*. Both types of research are highly valued in the scientific community.

Basic research is especially useful for constructing new theories and modifying existing theories. *Theories* are general explanations that attempt to explain the relationship between observable events (effects) and their origins (causes). Applied research is much narrower in scope but answers important questions of immediate social and clinical relevance. Applied research attempts to solve problems that require immediate solutions. However, basic research is often an impetus for finding solutions to practical problems. For example, Bloom's (1970) classic study of early language development was basic research—but it inspired many applied research studies and contributed much to the clinical domain.

Two types of applied research with distinctly different purposes are common in communication disorders. Olswang (1990) described the two distinct purposes as follows:

Applied research can be conducted for the purpose of better understanding the nature of communication disorders (i.e., exploring differences between normal and disordered populations), or for better understanding the clinical processes of assessment and treatment associated with communication disorders. (p. 45)

Applied research of the first type focuses on the nature of communication disorders, and any concern for immediate applications is secondary. Applied research of the second type is known as *clinical research*, and its primary purpose is to study some aspect of the clinical process. Clinical research may be further divided into special areas of interest such as assessment, treatment, or clinical specialties. The demand for clinical research is increased by needs for quality assurance, best practice, and evidence-based practice. Olswang (1990) explained as follows:

> Clinical research has been motivated in part by issues of accountability. Practitioners are asked to document the efficacy of their treatments, proving that what they do makes a difference in their clients' communicative functioning. Clinicians in school settings, health care settings, and private practice are asked to evaluate the efficacy of their services, to demonstrate that their efforts are worthwhile. (p. 45)

Laboratory and Field Studies

Another distinction in research types is between laboratory research and field research. *Field research* is conducted in everyday settings such as homes, schools, or clinics. In contrast, *laboratory research* is conducted in more or less contrived settings outside the mainstream of daily lives. Field research aims to observe behaviors as they occur in their natural environment. Field researchers may sacrifice close control over variables for closer ties to reality. In contrast, laboratory research maintains rigid control over variables but risks laboratory bias. In other words, laboratory surroundings may affect behavior in unwanted ways. For example, people who know they are being observed may change their behaviors in dramatic ways. Contemporary researchers have eliminated some of the unwanted effects of the laboratory environment to create laboratory settings that are remarkably natural.

Experimental and Quasi-Experimental Research Types

Experimental research is sometimes equated with laboratory research. However, many experiments are successfully conducted in field-like settings. Two requirements are central to the definition of a true experiment. First, participants are randomly assigned to two or more conditions. *Random assignment* of subjects to conditions assures *equivalency* and avoids the possibility of bias. Sometimes, researchers achieve near equivalency by *matching* subjects in Condition A with those in Condition B, but random assignment is the only way to assure equivalency. Second, researchers control the selection of conditions, and they can freely manipulate the conditions. If a research design does not meet these requirements, it is probably a *quasi-experimental* design.

The majority of designs in communication disorders research are classified as quasi-experimental. The prefix *quasi* means *as if, almost or having a likeness to.* Thus, quasi-experiments are almost experiments but not quite. Trochim (2004) described a quasi-experimental design as one that looks like an experimental design but lacks the key ingredient of random assignment.

Examples of true experiments in communication disorders are relatively few in number. A case example of a true experiment is Roy, Weinrich, Gray, Tanner, Stemple, and Sapienza's (2003) study of three treatments for teachers with voice disorders. The research team described the experimental protocol as follows:

> This randomized clinical trial used patient-based treatment outcome measures to evaluate the effectiveness of three treatment programs. Sixty-four teachers with voice disorders were randomly assigned to 1 of 3 treatment groups: voice amplification using the ChatterVox portable amplifier (VA; n = 25), resonance therapy (RT; n = 19), and respiratory muscle training (RMT; n = 20). Before and after a 6-week treatment phase, all teachers completed (a) the Voice Handicap Index (VHI; B. H. Jacobson et al., 1997), an instrument designed to appraise the self-perceived psychosocial consequences of voice disorders, and (b) a voice severity self-rating scale. (Roy et al., 2003, p. 670)

Based on the Roy et al. (2003) description, what qualifies the research design as a true experiment? How many conditions were employed in the experiment? In what way did the researchers control the selection of conditions?

Quasi-experimental research is divided into subcategories, each with distinctive features. The subcategories include: (a) correlational research, (b) developmental research, (c) survey research, (d) time-series designs, (e) historical research, and (f) comparative research. In quasi-experimental designs, important variables are typically observed after the fact of their existence.

For example, a study comparing severely hearing-impaired and mildly hearing-impaired persons investigates the effect of hearing impairment after the incident of hearing loss is well established. This is an example of a *nonequivalent groups design*—the most commonly employed research design in communication disorders.

Examples of nonequivalent-groups designs are plentiful in the communication disorders literature because clinical groups are often compared to nonclinical groups which serve as *controls*. Hoffman and Gillam (2004) described their nonequivalent groups of specific language-impaired (SLI) children and typically developing children as follows:

> The group of children with SLI contained 18 boys and 6 girls who ranged in age from 96 months to 128 months, with a mean age of 9;5 [. . .]. All children in the SLI group had been previously diagnosed as language impaired by public school assessment teams that included, at a minimum, a speech-language pathologist, a psychological examiner, and a classroom teacher, and all were receiving speech-language services in school at the time of the study. [. . .] The control group also contained 18 boys and 6 girls. They ranged in age from 96 to 128 months of age, with a mean age of 9:4 (see Table 1). Participants in the control group were selected on the basis of age, grade, and gender. Like their SLI counterparts, these children demonstrated normal hearing and nonverbal intelligence. Unlike their SLI counterparts, however, these children had no prior history of speech, language, or learning disorders. (pp. 117–118)

Though the children in Hoffman and Gillam's (2004) quasi-experiment were not exactly equivalent, the researchers attempted to establish some equivalency between the two groups. How did Hoffman and Gillam (2004) attempt to match the SLI and typically developing groups of children? In what ways were the two groups of children different?

Table 1.1   Common Threats to Internal Validity in Communication Disorders
Research, Most Vulnerable Research Designs, and Possible Remedies (Controls).

Threat	Vulnerable Design	Remedy (Control)
1. Ambiguous temporal precedence	Correlational and longitudinal designs	Choose another design if cause–effect is critical
2. Differential selection effect	Designs with two or more groups	(a) Randomly assign subjects to groups; (b) Match subjects
3. History effect	Observations over an extended time period	(a) Shorten length of experimental treatment
4. Maturation effect	(a) Lengthy experimental treatment (b) Complicated experimental task	(a) Shorten time of experimental treatment (b) Add control group to account for maturity effect
5. Statistical regression effect	Subjects selected on basis of high or low test scores	Deselect subjects with high or low test scores
6. Attrition effect	(a) Vulnerable subject population (b) Small sample size	Select additional subjects to offset losses
7. Testing effect	Subjects tested more than once during an experiment	(a) Counterbalance tests (b) Incorporate a time interval to extinguish effect
8. Instrument effect	Use of mechanical or electronic instruments; human observers (judges)	(a) Frequent calibration (b) Training (c) Perceptual anchors

A third case example is Tyler, Lewis, Haskill, and Tolbert's (2003) study of phonological and morphosyntactic changes in young children. Tyler et al. (2003) described their method as follows:

> Participants included 47 preschoolers, ages 3;0 (years; months) to 5;11, with impairments in both speech and language development: 40 children in the experimental group and 7 in a control group. All children had received speech-language evaluations and were identified as potential participants through review of their evaluation results in consultation with the evaluating SLP. Children in the experimental group were enrolled in speech-language services in early childhood programs in Washoe County School District, Reno, NV. For these children, speech-language services consisted of participation in one of the four experimental interventions. The control group consisted of children who had been placed on waiting lists for speech-language services. (p. 1079)

How should the Tyler et al. research be evaluated? What were the experimental conditions? What features make the design quasi-experimental? Could the researchers have employed random assignment of subjects to conditions? If the experiment was repeated, what could be done differently?

Types of Variables in Communication Disorders Research

Variables are the focus of interest for behavioral scientists. Variables are concepts that take on different quantitative or qualitative values. The opposite of a variable is known as a *constant.* Constants do not change—and they are not evident in human behavior. Examples of variables include *intelligence,* which has many values, and *gender,* which has two values—male and female. Thus, variables can have as few as two values or an infinite number of values. There are many different types of variables, but a critical distinction exists between those known as independent and dependent variables.

Independent and Dependent Variables. Independent and dependent variables are the focus of interest in research designs. In experimental research designs, researchers control and manipulate the independent variable, but in quasi-experimental designs, researchers cannot control or manipulate the independent variable because it is fixed. For example, Reynolds, Callihan, and Browning (2003) chose two forms of intervention (rhyming and narrative treatments) for 16 participants. The research team purposefully manipulated the independent variable by choosing two treatment conditions and randomly assigning half of the 16 participants to each of the two conditions. Reynolds et al. (2003) actively manipulated their independent variable, but many research designs include independent variables that cannot be manipulated. A case in point is McHenry's (2003) study of individuals with: (a) mild dysarthria, (b) moderate-to-severe dysarthria, and (c) no dysarthria (normal controls). In McHenry's quasi-experiment, the independent variable (dysarthric speech) was present before the study began and could not be manipulated by the researcher.

A second variable of central importance to research is known as the *dependent variable.* The dependent variable is the focus of observations in an experiment. It is usually a behavior that has been operationally defined. In experimental research, a relational hypothesis is typically written as a conditional statement: *if X, then Y.* In this form, *X* is the independent variable, and *Y* is the dependent variable. This is true for *bivariate research* problems that include one independent variable and one dependent variable. However, some experiments are designed to investigate *multivariate problems*—those that include more than one independent variable or more than one dependent variable. In multivariate research designs, the relational hypothesis is expressed as: *if X, then P and Q; or if P and Q, then Y.*

Active and Attribute Variables. Another important distinction made in research is one between active and attribute variables. *Active variables* are those that can be manipulated by the researcher. Examples of active variables include types of language tests, treatment procedures, noise, and other conditions that are readily changed. In contrast, *attribute variables* are measured but not manipulated. Human characteristics are attribute variables. Examples of attribute variables include language skills, intelligence, and hearing sensitivity. The assumption is that past environmental or hereditary incidents are responsible for these attributes; however, identifying exact causes is not always possible.

Continuous and Categorical Variables. A distinction between continuous and categorical variables is important for the preparation and analysis of research data. *Continuous variables* take on a range of values and possess the mathematical property known as *order*. For example, language age, chronological age, IQ, and hearing sensitivity are usually treated as continuous variables. In contrast, *categorical variables* do not have the mathematical property of *order*. In this case, people or objects are assigned to categories based on whether they possess some characteristic or not. Categorical variables may be dichotomous with only two values, or they may possess many values. For example, *gender* includes the categories male and female, but *hearing loss* may have five or more categories ranging from mild to profound. The number of categories depends on the classification scheme adopted by the researchers.

Artificial categories are sometimes created from continuous variables. For example, chronological age is clearly a continuous variable. However, age categories such as *young, middle-aged, old,* and *very old* are often constructed. To be meaningful, each category requires an *operational definition*. For example, the category *very old* may be operationally defined as 80 years of age and over. The important point is that categories can be created from continuous variables, and these newly created categories are treated as categorical variables. The use of variables in research designs will determine their classification as either continuous or categorical.

Extraneous Variables in Communication Disorders Research. In general, variables other than the independent variables and the dependent variables are unwanted and are often a nuisance in research. *Extraneous variables* are potential nuisance variables. In research, an extraneous variable is any variable that affects the dependent variable that is not the independent variable. If the dependent variable is affected by one or more extraneous variables, the relationship between independent and dependent variables is confounded. In this case, conclusions about the relationship between the independent and dependent variables are seriously compromised.

Extraneous variables are a regular occurrence and a persistent concern for researchers. They are particularly problematic in some research designs. However, if researchers are able to identify potential nuisance variables before a study begins, their effects may be minimized.

Operational Definitions in Communication Disorders Research

Research data are systematically collected and recorded according to guidelines (operational definitions) that are adopted by researchers during the early planning stages of experimentation. *Operational definitions* describe the activities necessary to measure and manipulate variables. More specifically, operational definitions are instructions for selecting subjects, measuring behaviors, and carrying out procedures.

Two Types of Operational Definitions. There are two types of operational definitions. One type specifies what behaviors will be measured. For example, a definition of stuttering lists the specific behaviors that the researcher believes represent the concept of stuttering. An operational definition is a bridge between concepts such as stuttering and observations such as syllable repetitions. Mizuko and Reichle (1989) adopted an operational definition for selecting participants based on specific behaviors. Their selection criteria were as follows:

> Subjects selected for the study met the following criteria: (a) English spoken as the primary language in the home, as reported by the subject's ward; (b) no apparent secondary handicaps—either physical, sensory (auditory or visual), or emotional—as reported by the subject's ward; (c) vision within normal limits, as determined by the Child's Recognition and Near Point Test (Allen, 1957); (d) hearing within normal limits, as determined by a pure-tone audiometric screening; (e) age equivalent scores between 2 and 5 years ($M = 3.19$ years; $SD = 0.73$), as determined by the Peabody Picture Vocabulary Test (Dunn, 1981); and (f) lack of familiarity with any of the three symbol systems, as determined by parental or teacher report. (Mizuko & Reichle, 1989, p. 628)

A second type of operational definition describes the manipulation of an independent variable. The independent variable in Mizuko and Reichle's (1989) study was the *graphic symbol system*. They selected three symbol systems as the experimental conditions—*Blissymbols, Picture Communication System,* and *Picsyms.* Mizuko and Reichle's (1989) operational definition included a description of the three symbol systems, as well as reasons for choosing them as follows:

> The rationale for selecting these symbol systems was twofold. First, these systems have been the focus of investigations with intellectually normal children (Mizuko, 1987). Second, one or more of these three symbol systems had been the focus of intervention studies with persons having moderate to severe handicaps (Goosens', 1983; Hurlbut et al., 1982; Leonhart & Maharaj, 1979). (p. 628)

The Limits of Operational Definitions.   Some variables are easily measured such as *gender* or *social class*. However, concepts like *intelligence* are more difficult to define. Any one or a combination of behaviors could form a definition of intelligence. In practice, researchers often rely on standardized measures of intelligence because they are reasonably objective and repeatable. Thus, a widely accepted test such as the *Stanford-Binet Intelligence Scale* is a common basis for operational definitions of intelligence. Likewise, researchers may choose a proven measure of hearing sensitivity or language ability for an operational definition. It is important that the measure chosen has been demonstrated to be both valid and reliable for the population of interest. What are examples of widely accepted tests for hearing sensitivity and language ability? Are they valid and reliable tests for the populations of children or adults that you treat?

Research Data in Communication Disorders

Research data are the consequence of observing or otherwise gathering information for study. Observations become data when they are coded in some fashion. These *codings* may take the form of written records or taped recordings. If the coding is not initially in numerical form, it is usually recoded numerically to facilitate data analysis. The assignment of numerals to objects according to specified rules is known as *measurement*. The data are also known as *statistics*. The science of statistics includes four steps: (a) collection, (b) classification, (c) analysis, and (d) interpretation of numerical data. The classification, analysis, and interpretation steps are faulty if data are not gathered in a reliable fashion.

The Reliability of Collected Data

The collection of data is a critical aspect of the scientific method and is a highly systematic process. Researchers must have a plan for gathering data that insures both objectivity and repeatability. Care must be taken to avoid personal biases in the collection of data that may unfairly affect the data. For example, a researcher who hypothesizes improved voice quality following treatment may unwittingly rate voice quality as better than it is in reality. Procedures for ensuring the reliability and validity of data collection include: (a) *interobserver reliability*, and (b) *blinding procedures*.

Blinding is the process of collecting data and performing other tasks prescribed by the research plan without knowledge of the research questions or hypotheses. To implement blinding procedures, researchers may recruit independent operatives to collect data and implement treatments. In the context of experimental research designs, *single blinding* is such that subjects do not know to which group they are assigned—experimental or control. In the case of *double blinding*, neither subjects nor research team members know who is assigned to experimental and control groups. Blinding is an important procedure in both experimental and quasi-experimental designs. It helps to insure the integrity of the research process.

Interobserver reliability is established by measuring the consistency of two or more individuals who independently observe the same event. The agreement between individuals is typically expected to be 90% or more depending on the exact nature of the observations. By convention, an *agreement index* below 80% is usually unacceptable. Interobserver agreement indexes are widely used to estimate the reliability of observational data. Two common computations for interobserver agreement are: (a) the *total percentage agreement* (also known as the *smaller/larger index*) and (b) the *point-by-point agreement*.

The total percentage agreement procedure is calculated for two sets of scores by dividing the smaller number of behaviors observed by the larger number. For example, Observer A records 22 occurrences of a behavior, and Observer B records 18 occurrences. To calculate the percentage of agreement, the 18 is divided by 22 to equal 0.82. The result is converted to a percentage by multiplying 0.82 by 100. The result is an 82% agreement between observers. This procedure assumes that the two sets of scores overlap. In other words, Observer A identified the same 18 occurrences of the behavior as Observer B plus 4 additional occurrences. When this assumption is not met, an alternative procedure such as the point-by-point agreement index is employed.

The point-by-point agreement index is a common interobserver agreement metric in communication disorders. This procedure examines targeted behaviors point-by-point as shown in the table below. The symbol 0 represents the absence of a target behavior, and

1 represents its presence. A point-by-point inspection of the data reveals two points of disagreement between Observers A and B with a total of eight points of agreement.

Observer A	Observer B	
1	0	disagree
1	1	agree
0	0	agree
1	1	agree
1	1	agree
0	0	agree
1	1	agree
0	1	disagree
0	0	agree
1	1	agree

Thus, 8 divided by 10 (total points of comparison) yields a coefficient of 0.80. The result is converted to a percentage by multiplying 0.80 by 100 for an 80% agreement between observers. This procedure is generally a good index of interobserver reliability.

Internal Validity in Communication Disorders Research

The concept of *internal validity* was first introduced by Campbell (1957). Internal validity is the minimum requirement for meaningful interpretations of research results. Internal validity is the degree to which the relationship between the independent variable (IV) and dependent variable (DV) is observed without the influence of extraneous variables. If there is a causal inference, the relationship is hypothesized as IV → DV. Variables that affect the DV other than the IV are known as *confounding* (or extraneous) variables. The presence of confounding variables weakens internal validity. As a consequence, when internal validity is weak, researchers cannot imply that the IV produced the effect observed in the DV. Problems with internal validity are the most common weakness in research studies.

Campbell and Stanley (1963) described eight common threats to internal validity, including: (a) differential selection effects, (b) history effects, (c) maturation effects, (d) statistical regression effects, (e) attrition effects, (f) testing effects, (g) instrumentation effects, and (h) additive and interaction effects. These are sometimes referred to as the eight classic threats. Shadish, Cook, and Campbell (2002) added another threat, *ambiguous temporal precedence,* to the list of common threats to internal validity. Thus, nine common threats to internal validity are important considerations for researchers as they plan their investigations in communication disorders. However, the nine threats do not affect every research design. Rather, some designs are more vulnerable to certain threats—and some are less vulnerable.

Ambiguous Temporal Precedence Effects.   To infer causality, the treatment must occur before a change in the dependent variable is observed. However, the direction of a relationship between two variables is not always clear. When the direction of relationship between two variables is uncertain, the relationship is best described as $A \leftrightarrow B$. Correlational and longitudinal designs are especially vulnerable to *ambiguous temporal precedence* (ATP) effects because the temporal relationship between variables is often ambiguous.

Controlling ATP Effects.   There are no specific procedures for controlling ATP effects. Rather, the only way to avoid the threat of ATP effects is to choose a research design that is not vulnerable to such effects, such as pretest–posttest designs. However, if causality is not important to the research purpose, ATP effects are not a concern. Why are pretest-posttest designs immune to ATP effects?

Differential Selection Effects.   The participants in research studies possess unique characteristics (learned and inherent), such as gender, age, intelligence, culture, and motor skills. Research designs that employ two or more groups of participants are especially vulnerable to differential selection threats. If subjects are assigned to experimental and control groups in a way that results in an unequal distribution of the subjects' unique characteristics, differential selection is a serious threat. The results from such an experiment are confounded. If there is a difference between groups, the difference may be caused by the independent variable effect, or by the subject-related effect.

Controlling Selection Effects.   In the case of research designs with one subject or one group of subjects, selection effects are not a problem. The best way to control selection effects is to randomly assign subjects to experimental and control groups. *Random assignment* of subjects to groups usually avoids differential selection effects. In research designs in which two or more groups of subjects are compared, an important assumption is that the groups are homogeneous in all respects. In quasi-experimental designs, the groups are homogeneous except for the classification variable. The classification variable is the one feature that distinguishes one group from the other. For example, research in communication disorders often includes groups that are distinguished by clinical classifications, such as persons with cochlear implants. To minimize the effects of differential selection in research designs where random assignment to groups is impossible, *matching* procedures are employed. If properly implemented, matching procedures ensure that the groups are equivalent for critical features, such as intelligence, age, gender, culture, or others. What other characteristics (learned or inherent) may be especially important as matching criteria?

History Effects.   History effects include outside events (extraneous variables) that may influence the dependent variable during the course of a study. Research designs that require observations over long periods of time are especially vulnerable to the threat of history effects. The observations in comparative studies are sometimes accomplished in a few days, so they are less vulnerable to history effects. In contrast, longitudinal designs are especially vulnerable because of the duration of time involved. Pretest–posttest designs may or may not be especially vulnerable, depending on the duration of time between pretest and posttest phases. What are some extraneous variables that could produce a history effect in an experiment with children who are observed over the course of 3 months?

Controlling History Effects.   History problems are managed by anticipating their occurrence and controlling their effect. If a research plan requires a lengthy period of treatment or observations, the opportunity for extraneous variables to interfere is high. However, a research plan that accomplishes an experimental protocol in two or three weeks will probably avoid confounding by history effects. If researchers identify an extraneous variable but are unable to avoid its effect, they may choose to eliminate its effect at the experiment's conclusion with the help of special statistical procedures. However, statistical control of an extraneous variable is only possible if the variable is measured.

Maturation Effects.   Students sometimes confuse history and maturation effects. Maturation effects include changes within the organism, not outside events. Examples include changes in physical abilities and mental processes such as children's development of speech and language or motor skills. In the special case of adults with aphasia, *time postonset* is a variable that may produce a maturation effect. Brookshire (1983) explained as follows:

> This information is particularly important when subjects' participation in an experiment spans several days or weeks, because if short-time postonset subjects who are in a period of neurologic recovery are included, changes in their responses during the course of the experiment may reflect the effects of neurologic recovery, rather than the effects of experimental conditions. (p. 343)

In addition to longer-term maturation effects, shorter-term maturation effects such as boredom, fatigue, and inattention are risks for maturation effects. Experimental tasks that are long or complicated may produce maturation effects such as boredom and fatigue, and these factors can significantly affect the dependent variable. As a case example, Tharpe and Ashmead (2001) reported a longitudinal study of seven infants. They measured auditory sensitivity monthly from birth to 12 months of age. *Maturation* was the independent variable as is typical in developmental research, so the maturation effect was the focus of the study. Were there any *history effects* that may have affected the dependent variable (auditory sensitivity)?

Controlling Maturation Effects.   Maturation effects are minimized by reducing the time required for completing observations, however, shortening an experiment's length is not always possible. An alternative is the addition of a control group that is expected to mature at the same rate as the experimental group. Because the control group does not receive the experimental treatment, a difference between the groups may be attributed to the treatment effect. Short-term maturation effects may be controlled by modifying the experimental milieu in ways that minimize boredom, fatigue, and inattention. For example, planned rest periods or more comfortable surroundings may reduce fatigue and improve attention for some participants. What other preventive measures could be employed to avoid maturation effects, both short- and long-term?

Statistical Regression Effects.   Statistical regression predicts that subjects who score very high or very low on a test tend to regress toward the mean on the next administration of the test. For example, high scores tend to move lower and low scores tend to move higher. As a case example, if participants score 10% on a speech discrimination test, they will probably score higher on the next administration of the test. Statistical regression effects are a threat to internal validity when subjects are assigned to groups or conditions based on extreme scores (high or low) on a test. A subsequent change in the dependent variable may be attributed to the treatment effect or statistical regression (extraneous variable).

Controlling Statistical Regression Effects.   Statistical regression effects are minimized by not selecting subjects based on extreme test scores. For example, subjects who participate in pretest–posttest research designs can be deselected if their pretest score is extremely high or low. However, deselecting subjects presents a threat to internal validity of another kind—*attrition effects.*

Attrition Effects.   Attrition effects (also known as mortality effects) involve a loss of participants because of one or more reasons. For example, subjects may drop out of a study for unknown reasons, or subjects may relocate to another geographic area. Another possibility is that subjects cease to meet selection criteria because of physical changes, mental changes, or extreme scores on a pretest measure. Studies that require a long period of time for completion are especially vulnerable to attrition effects. Developmental studies are especially vulnerable because they typically require many months or years for completion. Some populations are especially vulnerable to attrition effects due to chronic illnesses and other health-related characteristics. What are some other possible sources of attrition?

Controlling Attrition Effects.   It is sometimes difficult to anticipate the loss of participants. However, researchers should plan for attrition based on the characteristics of participants and length of the study. When attrition is expected, researchers can avoid attrition effects by selecting additional participants to offset possible losses.

Testing Effects.   If subjects are tested more than once during an experiment, *multiple-test effects* are possible. Testing effects occur when one test affects performance on a second test. The result may be: (a) a test-sensitizing effect, (b) a test-practice effect, or (c) a combination of the two effects. *Test-sensitizing effects* are changes in the subjects' anxiety levels in anticipation of test taking. Anxiety usually abates after the first test, and performance on the second test improves. However, test anxiety may increase after the first test, particularly if the subject initially perceives the test as very difficult. *Test-practice effects* are the result of acquiring specific skills that improve performance on the second test. Test-sensitizing and test-practice effects are especially troublesome in research designs with two or more administrations of the same test.

Controlling Testing Effects.   The method of *counterbalancing* tests is often employed to control testing effects. For example, half the subjects take Test A followed by Test B; the other half take Test B followed by Test A. In this fashion, the halves are averaged, and the adverse testing effects are minimized. An alternative is to plan an interval of time between tests to extinguish testing effects.

Instrumentation Effects.   The threat of instrumentation effects has to do with unwanted variations in instruments used to measure human behaviors. Researchers may use mechanical or electronic devices to collect data, or they may employ human observers. Both mechanical instruments and human vary because of internal fluctuations and external influences. Mechanical and electronic equipment may change over time in response to temperature, humidity, jarring, and mechanical wear. Human observers may change over time because of distractions, inattentiveness, or physical discomforts.

Controlling Instrument Effects.   Mechanical and electronic instruments require frequent calibrations to ensure consistent measurements. Human observers may benefit from training to minimize the variability in their observations and judgments. For example, *perceptual anchors* usually minimize variability when rating scales are employed as observational tools. Perceptual anchors are typically auditory or visual models that serve to establish the upper and lower limits of a rating scale. In addition to training and perceptual anchors as controls, researchers may employ observers who are experts by virtue of prior training, experience, and credentials that are relevant to the study's purpose.

Additive and Interaction Effects.   One or more of the many potential threats to internal validity may interact with one another. For example, selection effects often interact with maturation, history, or instrumentation effects. The direction and size of additive and interaction effects are not readily identified or measured. There are no controls for additive and interaction effects except eliminating threats to internal validity when possible and minimizing the threats that are identified but unavoidable. How might selection effects interact with maturation, history, or instrumentation effects?

External Validity in Communication Disorders Research

External validity refers to the generalizability of research results to other participants and settings. This is an especially important consideration for transferring research results to clinical practice. Threats to external validity are of two types. One is known as threats to *population validity*—problems with generalization to other people. The other is known as threats to *ecological validity*—problems with generalization to other environments (Bracht & Glass, 1968). Seven factors may limit the ability to generalize research results to other persons and settings. The first limitation concerns *accessible populations* and *target populations*.

Accessible Populations and Target Populations.   Target populations are the entire populations that are of interest to researchers. For example, researchers may be interested in American-born, 12-year-old children with Down syndrome. The total population with these characteristics includes a large number of children distributed throughout the country and elsewhere. Accessible populations include all people who can be participants given the researchers' available resources. Many researchers are limited to recruiting participants from a restricted locale such as a city, state, or region. In this case, generalization of results is usually restricted to the accessible population. A case example is Walden, Surr, Cord, and Dyrlund's (2004) study of hearing aid microphone preferences in everyday listening situations. The research team recruited participants (16 males, 1 female) from the accessible population of hearing-impaired adults with hearing aids fitted at the Walter Reed Army Medical Center. In this case, what is the ability to generalize to other persons and other settings?

Describing the Independent Variable Explicitly.   The procedures followed by researchers must be described in sufficient detail to be duplicated in other settings. Detailed descriptions of procedures are especially important if results are to be generalized to clinical practice settings.

Multiple-Treatment Interference Effects.   If participants receive more than one treatment consecutively, the external validity of subsequent treatments is uncertain—because the subsequent treatment may have reacted to the initial treatment. Thus, the effects of subsequent treatments may not be generalizable to situations without the benefit of a preceding treatment.

Novelty and Disruption Effects.   "A new and unusual experimental treatment, e.g., a [teaching] innovation, may be superior to a traditional treatment primarily because it is novel" (Bracht & Glass, 1968). In other words, the difference between treatments may disappear when the novelty is gone. A different kind of effect is known as a *disruption effect*. The treatment effect is disrupted because researchers are less skillful in their administration of a new and unfamiliar treatment. Thus, the new treatment may be less effective than the traditional treatment. A familiarization routine before a study begins may reduce the novelty effect—and practice will minimize the disruption effect.

Experimenter Effects.   Researchers may unintentionally affect the behaviors of participants. Experimenter effects are typically associated with: (a) differences in the researchers' behavior—such as mannerisms or verbal reinforcements, (b) the researchers' appearances—such as clothing, gender, or age, and (c) bias in the researchers' observations and recording of data. Experimenter effects are minimized by insuring that researchers interact with participants in a uniform manner. Biases in observations and the recording of data are minimized by employing independent observers and utilizing blinding procedures.

Pretest and Posttest Sensitization Effects.   The experimental effect may be confounded by the presence of pretest or posttest administrations. Pretest and posttest sensitization effects limit the generalization of results to those situations where the pretest or posttest is also present. The use of unobtrusive measures minimizes the effect of pretests and posttests.

Measurement of the Dependent Variable.   The operational definition of the dependent variable may limit generalization and transferability of results to clinical practice settings. For example, if a dependent variable such as cognitive development is operationally defined by a series of Piagetian tasks—the research results may not generalize to cognitive development that is measured in other ways.

Conclusion: Scientific Inquiry in Communication Disorders Research

The *literature* (body of research reports) in communication sciences and disorders is rich with examples of scientific inquiry, including a wide range of designs, methods, and topics of interest. The published articles provide opportunities to evaluate methods and to acquire ideas for research and clinical practice. A case in point is Stewart, Pankiw, Lehman, and Simpson's (2002) report of hearing in users of recreational firearms. Their purpose was to determine hearing loss and hearing handicap for shooters. To recruit participants, Stewart et al. (2002) approached customers as they entered a sporting goods store the weekend before deer hunting season. The research team asked customers to participate in the study. The 232 volunteers (45 females, 187 males) were also given a $5 gift certificate for the purchase of any item in the sporting goods store as an incentive. The subjects completed short questionnaires to collect demographic data and information about firearm use. The research team subsequently obtained hearing thresholds in a mobile hearing unit with sound booths. Participants who were identified with hearing loss ≥ 25 dB ($n = 177$) completed the *Hearing Handicap Inventory for Adults*.

Stewart et al. (2002) found that males, older individuals, and blue-collar workers exhibited more high-frequency hearing loss and more hearing handicap than others. Based on what you know about the Stewart et al. (2002) study, answer the following questions:

1. What is your evaluation of the method for recruiting subjects?
2. What threats to internal validity may have been present in the study?
3. What is your evaluation of the study's external validity?
4. What was the target population?
5. What was the accessible population?
6. If the study is replicated, in what way would you change the method?
7. How are the results useful for clinical practice?

For students, teachers, and clinicians who have a special interest in research, plentiful examples of research are found in the scholarly journals—including journals published by the American Speech-Language-Hearing Association (ASHA), the American Academy of Audiology (AAA), and the National Student Speech Language Hearing Association (NSSLHA). The various journals sponsored by these professional associations are as follows:

1. The *Journal of Speech, Language, and Hearing Research* pertains broadly to studies of the processes and disorders of speech, language, and hearing, and to the diagnosis and treatment of such disorders (American Speech-Language-Hearing Association, 2004).
2. The *American Journal of Audiology: A Journal of Clinical Practice* pertains to all aspects of clinical practice in audiology (American Speech-Language-Hearing Association, 2004).
3. The *American Journal of Speech-Language Pathology: A Journal of Clinical Practice* pertains to all aspects of clinical practice in speech-language pathology (American Speech-Language-Hearing Association, 2004).

4. *Language, Speech, and Hearing Services in Schools* pertains to speech, hearing, and language services for children and adolescents, particularly in schools (American Speech-Language-Hearing Association, 2004).
5. *Contemporary Issues in Communication Science and Disorders* pertains to diverse issues in speech, language, and hearing of special interest to students (National Student Speech Language Hearing Association, 2004).
6. The *Journal of the American Academy of Audiology* pertains to diverse issues in audiology (American Academy of Audiology, 2004b).

CASE STUDIES

Case 1.1   Snooping for Unusual Data

You collected the following pretest data for 12 participants. Is there a problem with the data? How should you proceed?

54	49
13	50
61	60
67	60
44	50
89	46

Case 1.2   Nuisance Variables for Professor Ross?

Professor Ross and you are planning a follow-up study to determine the speech outcomes for 20 students that you treated for pervasive /s/ problems when they were in elementary school. The former students are between 13 and 21 years of age. What internal validity problems do you anticipate?

Case 1.3   Question of Time

You begin an investigation of treatment outcomes for 10 adults with aphasia, but the participants' post-onset times are varied. Is there a threat to internal validity? How should you proceed with the study?

Post-Onset	Time (weeks)
8	20
52	24
12	48
50	51
58	60

Student Exercises

1. Physical dimensions are easily measured because there are natural units of measurement—such as inches or pounds. However, psychological variables are not easily measured because they lack natural units of measurement. This is a problem for *construct validity*. What is your operational definition for the construct known as *language development?*

2. Review one issue from a contemporary journal in communication disorders. How many research articles in the issue include one or more research questions? How many statements of hypotheses can you find?

3. Locate a research report on a topic of interest in communication disorders. What *participant selection criteria* were specified by the researchers? What is the population of interest that the sample represents? What is the level of generalization for the research results?

4. Examine the Methods section of a research article in communication disorders. What are the procedures and what instruments were used by the researchers? Did the researchers employ *blinding procedures?*

5. Locate a research article in communication disorders. What *operational definitions* were included in the Methods section of the report? Evaluate the researchers' operational definitions. Are the definitions valid ones?

2 Ethics in Communication Disorders Research

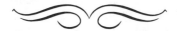

eth·ic   (eth ′ik) *n.* belief, conduct, conscience, convention, criterion, decency, goodness, honesty, honor, ideal, imperative, integrity, morality, practice, principle, standard, value.

Research ethics are rules of conduct that are usually based on a history of sound and logical research practice. Ethical standards are not intended to slow the progress of science. Instead, they should encourage honesty in reporting data, accuracy in describing procedures, and fairness in the treatment of research participants. Matters of ethical conduct are inseparable from matters of research design because some designs are more likely to cause discomfort or harm to participants. Thus, ethical decision making is accomplished during the initial planning process for research.

A Brief History of Research Ethics

The impetus for formalizing rules of conduct in experimentation and research comes from a long history of human rights abuses. Accounts of human rights abuses for the sake of experimentation are present in the earliest recorded history. During the 1st century B.C., the Egyptian queen, Cleopatra, speculated that gestation periods were different for females and males. To test the hypothesis, she ordered her handmaids impregnated and their wombs opened at specified times to observe fetal development firsthand—an abomination of human rights. Another example of human rights abuse occurred near the end of the 19th century when Dr. Arthur Wentworth performed spinal taps on 29 children at Children's Hospital of Boston. He hypothesized that the procedure was harmless. At the experiment's conclusion, Dr. Wentworth pronounced the surgical procedure painful but harmless. The experiment may have provided some new information for medical science—but its

23

participants suffered intolerable abuse. Dr. Wentworth was subsequently reprimanded by his colleagues and widely criticized by others.

An atrocity of human rights abuse with official sanctions was perpetrated in 1932. In that year, the United States Public Health Service began a longitudinal study of untreated syphilis with more than 400 African-American men in Tuskegee, Alabama. The study continued for 40 years while available medical treatments were withheld from participants. In remarks at the White House in 1997, President Clinton apologized to survivors and relatives: "The people who ran the study at Tuskegee diminished the stature of man by abandoning the most basic ethical precepts" (*White House OPS*, 1997). Speech-language pathology has suffered lapses in research ethics as well.

It was 1939 when Professor Wendell Johnson and a graduate student (Mary Tudor) attempted to increase disfluencies in two groups of children: (a) stutterers, and (b) normally-fluent children. The participants in the *Tudor Study* were children living in a state-supported orphanage. Johnson and Tudor deceived the children and misled the orphanage's staff. Furthermore, they made no attempt to *debrief* the children or the children's caretakers when the study concluded. A reexamination of the Tudor Study's results suggested that the experiment caused an unpleasant reaction in some of the children but no lasting affect (Ambrose & Yairi, 2002). Nonetheless, the procedures employed by Johnson and Tudor are unacceptable by today's standards. Though contemporary researchers have adopted basic ethical principles, isolated cases of abuse continue to surface.

The rights of individuals have been debated since the earliest annals of recorded history. The ethical principle, *primum non nocere* (first do no harm), was inspired by the Greek physician Hippocrates who lived in the 5th century B.C. In 1865, Claude Barnard, a French physiologist, published a book about human experimentation and admonished researchers as follows: "Never perform an experiment which might be harmful to the patient even though highly advantageous to science or the health of others." In 1947, in the aftermath of World War II, the Nuremberg Code was adopted. It addressed the importance of free choice in experimentation as follows: "The voluntary consent of the human subject is absolutely essential." In 1966, the *National Institutes of Health's Office for Protection of Research Subjects* issued a policy statement establishing independent research review bodies known as *Institutional Review Boards*.

The purpose of Institutional Review Boards (IRBs) is to independently review research plans and insure that participants are treated fairly. In 1979, the National Commission for the Protection of Human Subjects of Biomedical and Behavioral Research issued a statement titled *Ethical Principles and Guidelines for Research Involving Human Subjects* (*Belmont Report*). The *Belmont Report* was so named because the National Commission convened in the Smithsonian Institution's Belmont Conference Center. The National Commission accomplished three goals:

1. It distinguished between research and practice.
2. It identified three basic ethical principles.
3. It described applications for the three basic principles.

In regard to the third goal, the applications for the three basic principles described in the *Belmont Report* were: (a) *informed consent,* (b) *risk-benefit assessment,* and (c) *selection of*

Technology Note

The emergence of new technologies is a challenge for ethics in research as well as clinical practice. Technological advancements raise new questions about what is acceptable conduct in experimentation and other professional endeavors. For example, Meline and Mata-Pistokache (2003) addressed the hazards inherent in email technology. Technological innovations such as email are useful tools for research, but their emergence requires reexamining codes of ethical conduct. A related issue is the use of technology to extend audiology and speech-language pathology services across state boundaries (cf. Frazik, 2003). The *Digital Era Copyright Enhancement Act* (1999) addressed new legal issues stemming from advances in technology. Likewise, the American Speech-Language-Hearing Association's Board of Ethics published new guidelines to address the plagiarism dilemmas created by advances in technology (Ethics Board, 2002).

research participants. The *Belmont Report* is important because it is the framework for contemporary codes of professional conduct in research.

Professional Codes of Ethics and Research

Today, most researchers agree on a set of moral principles to guide the conduct of experimentation. However, new and changing technologies are a challenge for professional associations and state license boards, which are responsible for establishing standards for ethical conduct. The speech-language pathology and audiology professions are likely to adopt new technologies for their practices and research endeavors as they become available. The *California Occupation Guide* described speech-language pathology and audiology as *high-tech* professions:

> Future speech-language pathologists (SLPs) and audiologists will routinely use computers to screen the speech and language skills of students and adults with communication disabilities and to provide further diagnostic testing when needed. Clients in therapy can use programs between sessions that not only present stimuli, but evaluate responses and give immediate feedback automatically. (California Employment Development Department, 1995)

Technology affects methods for experimentation, as well as those for clinical interventions. Researchers are increasingly using the Internet for online experimentation, and chat rooms and email for collecting research data—raising new issues of privacy, confidentiality, and informed consent. The increased dependence on high-tech resources such as networked computers and the internet will probably require further examination of existing codes of conduct for researchers and clinicians.

The set of principles that guide the conduct of experimentation is formalized and written as a *code of ethics.* Organizations of physicians, psychologists, audiologists, speech-language pathologists, and others have adopted codes of ethics that address standards for acceptable behaviors (*prescriptions*) and unacceptable behaviors (*proscriptions*). Because members of professional organizations may engage in research activities in addition to clinical practice, codes of ethics usually include standards for research along with standards for clinical practice.

The *Belmont Report* recognized *practice* and *research* as distinctly different activities, though the two activities may overlap, such as in the case of research that aims to discover more effective therapy techniques. *Practice* refers to interventions with the sole purpose of improving the well-being of an individual client, or patient. On the other hand, *research* tests hypotheses, makes conclusions, and extends results to the population of interest. For research, the benefit to society as a whole may outweigh the well-being of individual participants. The *Belmont Report* identified three basic ethical principles: (a) respect for persons, (b) beneficence, and (c) justice.

Ethical Principle One: Respect for Persons

The principle of *respect for persons* requires researchers to recognize participants in experiments as persons of worth who participate by free choice. An application of this principle is called informed consent. The basic elements of an informed consent document are outlined in Table 2.1. Informed consent is the knowing consent of an individual or legally authorized representative who is able to exercise free choice without undue inducement, force, fraud, deceit, duress, constraint, or coercion (Korchin & Cowan, 1982). To meet the standard of respect, researchers must insure that participants are provided complete information about the experiment, participants understand the information, and participants are willing volunteers.

Ethical Principle Two: Beneficence

A second ethical principle that is identified in the *Belmont Report* is *beneficence*. Researchers should make every effort to insure the well-being of research participants. Researchers are expected to: (a) do no harm to participants, and (b) maximize benefits and minimize risks to participants. *Benefit* refers to something of positive value to participants, and *risk* refers to the possibility of harm to participants. Inhumane treatment of participants is never acceptable, and risks should never exceed the minimum necessary to achieve the research goals. Benefits should always outweigh risks in an analysis of risks and benefits.

Ethical Principle Three: Justice

A third ethical principle that is identified in the *Belmont Report* is *justice*. This principle is concerned with the equal treatment of people in society. It concerns the fair and equitable distribution of burdens and benefits. The Tuskegee study is an example of injustice because the burden was on African-American men—but syphilis affects people of all races and gender. The choice of research participants should be evaluated for possible selection biases. For example, participants may be selected because they are readily

Table 2.1   Basic Elements of a Consent Form

1. *Explanation of the Procedures*
   The purpose of the study and a description of the procedures should be included. The activity should be identified as research.

2. *Risks or Discomforts*
   Any foreseeable risks and discomforts to the participant should be described. Risks should be quantified if possible.

3. *Benefits*
   Expected benefits from the research to the participant or others should be described.

4. *Alternative Procedures*
   Alternative procedures or treatments that might be beneficial to the participant should be disclosed.

5. *Confidentiality*
   The degree of confidentiality should be described, including who will have access to the participant's records.

6. *Termination of Participation*
   Individuals should be informed that they are free to withdraw consent and discontinue participation in the research at any time without prejudice. In addition, circumstances under which the investigator may terminate their participation without their consent should be disclosed.

7. *Costs to Participants*
   Costs to individuals from participation in the study should be disclosed including no costs.

8. *Payment for Participation*
   Any amount or other payment to be paid to the subject for participation should be specified.

9. *Questions*
   An offer to answer any questions concerning the procedures along with a name and phone number of a person to contact should be included.

10. *Legal Rights*
    A statement indicating that the individual is not waiving any legal rights by signing the form should be included.

11. *Patient Initials*
    If the consent form has more than one page, a provision for initialing the first pages should be included.

12. *Signatures*
    A place for signatures of the participant, a witness, and dates of receipt should be included.

13. *Copy for Participant*
    A copy should be provided to the participant.

14. *Additional Elements for Research with Children*
    Children should be given an opportunity to consent or refuse participation. Their expression of consent or refusal should be indicated on the form. Signatures are expected for older children. Younger children may demonstrate consent in a variety of ways.

Note: A *waiver* may be appropriate if a child is not capable of indicating consent because of the child's mental state or chronological age. In every case, consent of at least one parent or legal guardian is required. If more than minimal risk is involved, both parents (legal guardians) should signify consent. Special provisions may be made for children who are wards of the state, an agency, or institution.

available—known as *samples of convenience*—or selected because of inherent vulnera-bilities. In the latter case, institutionalized persons, students, patients, immigrants, and the poor are especially vulnerable. The selection of participants should correspond closely to the purpose of the research.

Statements of Ethics in Research

The rules of conduct found in codes of ethics written by professional organizations are obligatory for their members. For example, the American Psychological Association (APA) addressed the issues of respect for persons, beneficence, and justice in *Ethical Principles of Psychologists and Code of Conduct* (American Psychological Association, 2002). The American Speech-Language-Hearing Association (ASHA) addressed the issues of respect for persons, beneficence, and justice in its *Code of Ethics* (2003). The pream-ble to ASHA's *Code of Ethics* includes "speech, language, and hearing scientists" as a group of individuals who are governed by the *Code*. The members of the American Speech-Language-Hearing Association are obliged to abide by the following rules of conduct re-garding research.

1. *Principle of Ethics I. (Preface)* Individuals shall honor their responsibility to hold para-mount the welfare of persons they serve professionally or participants in research and scholarly activities and shall treat animals involved in research in a humane manner. [*beneficence*]
2. *Principle of Ethics I. (Rules of Ethics C)* Individuals shall not discriminate in the delivery of professional services or the conduct of research and scholarly activities on the basis of race or ethnicity, gender, age, religion, national origin, sexual orientation, or disabil-ity. [*justice*]
3. *Principle of Ethics I. (Rules of Ethics F)* Individuals shall [. . .] inform participants in re-search about the possible effects of their participation in research conducted. [*respect for persons*]
4. *Principle of Ethics I. (Rules of Ethics N)* Individuals shall use persons in research or as subjects of teaching demonstrations only with their informed consent. [*respect for persons*]

The American Academy of Audiology (AAA) addressed issues of privacy, informed consent, and freedom of choice in the *Code of Ethics of the American Academy of Audiol-ogy (Rule 5d)*:

> *Code of Ethics of the American Academy of Audiology. (Rule 5d)* Individuals shall not carry out teaching or research activities in a manner that constitutes an invasion of privacy, or that fails to inform persons fully about the nature and possible effects of these activities, affording all persons informed free choice of participation (American Academy of Audiology, 2004a). [*respect for persons*]

State license laws and regulations for audiologists and speech-language pathologists may incorporate statements of ethics that specifically address research endeavors. For ex-ample, Illinois' *Professional Conduct Standards* specify the following behaviors as uneth-ical or unprofessional conduct:

> Failing to inform prospective research subjects or their authorized representative fully of po-tentially serious after effects of the research or failing to remove the after effects as soon as

the design of the research permits. (State of Illinois Division of Professional Regulations, 2004)

Issues in Research Ethics

Research Participants

Research plans typically include human subjects in their procedures. However, the term *subject* is not sufficient to include all the people who may participate in an experiment. The term *participant* is a better choice to describe individuals who have an active role in a research study. A research participant should be viewed as a partner or collaborator—not simply a cooperative subject (Korchin & Cowan, 1982). Research participants are not only those who receive a treatment, but they may be those individuals who assume supportive roles. For example, research studies sometimes include observers who are employed to judge a behavior or other event. These *judges* are considered to be participants in a study and are entitled to the same rights as other participants, such as informed consent.

Researchers choose participants for their studies based on their purpose and methodology. For example, a research report in the journal *Language, Speech, and Hearing Services in Schools* sought to investigate language-impaired children's social pretend play and conversational behaviors (Dekroon, Kyle, & Johnson, 2002). The researchers selected seven boys as participants. Three participants were language impaired and four were not. As a general principle, the choice of participants is expected to match the purpose of the study. In this case, it was not clear why the researchers selected only boys as subjects. On the other hand, a research report in the *American Journal of Audiology* included 191 women (no men) as participants (Erler & Garstecki, 2002). The Erler and Garstecki (2002) study's stated purpose was to determine whether women vary by age by the degree of stigma they attach to hearing loss and hearing aid use. In this case, the selection of women as participants closely matched the stated purpose of the research.

Distributive justice has to do with the inclusion or exclusion of research participants based on genuine needs and not based on social, racial, sexual, or cultural bias. An injustice occurs when researchers purposely exclude a class of people who may benefit from research or when researchers purposely include a class of people because of convenience or based on their vulnerabilities. There are classes of people, such as women and ethnic minorities, who may be excluded from research that could otherwise be beneficial to them. Likewise, certain classes of people, such as disadvantaged individuals, may be disproportionately included in research studies that contain significant risks. Researchers are encouraged to select participants carefully to avoid social injustices and to insure that the benefits of research are distributed fairly.

Informed Consent

There are many potential barriers to informed consent. Achieving the goal of informed consent is confounded when participants are especially vulnerable or unable to fully comprehend the information. This is a special problem for children, as well as adults with diminished cognitive abilities. For example, adults who are unable to make informed decisions, such as some individuals with aphasia or with Alzheimer's disease, are especially vulnerable.

Individuals who reside in institutions are sometimes recruited for participation in research studies. For example, a study reported in the *Journal of Speech and Hearing Disorders* included 272 prison inmates as participants (Walton, McCardle, Crowe, & Wilson, 1990). Though the participants signed an informed consent form prior to their participation in the study, they may or may not have been willing volunteers. Institutionalized persons, such as nursing home residents and prisoners, are especially vulnerable because of their dependency on others. What are other examples of persons who may be especially vulnerable?

To insure voluntary and informed consent with special populations, proxy consents may be sought from parents, custodians, or other responsible persons. However, parental consent or consent from others—no matter how well informed—is not sufficient to place a child or another vulnerable person in a potentially harmful experiment (*Court of Appeals of Maryland,* 2001).

Another barrier to informed consent is *comprehension*—or the lack of it. Nearly half the population in the Unites States reads at or below the 8th-grade level, and some Americans have little or no reading skills. In 1982, Korchin and Cowan reported that some consent documents require college-level reading ability. Today, readability remains an important issue because the language in consent forms is sometimes two or three grade levels above recommended reading levels (Paashe-Orlow, Taylor, & Brancati, 2003). The reading level for informed consent documents should be between the 6th- and 8th-grade levels, which is the reading level found in newspapers. However, the reading level should be adjusted accordingly for special populations. To insure readability, researchers can test their consent documents with several prospective participants from the target population before the experiment begins.

The following description was included in the Informed Consent Form for a study of the effects of vocal training on respiration, phonation, and articulation with participants ranging in age from 18 to 35 years:

Technology Note

The readability level of a passage can be checked by using a tool that is built into Microsoft Word. On the Tools menu, click Options, click the Spelling & Grammar tab, and check the box labeled Show readability statistics. Highlight the text to be analyzed and click on the Spelling and Grammar tab on the Tools menu to begin the readability analysis. The result is a list of readability statistics that includes the *Flesch Reading Ease* score and the *Flesch-Kincaid Grade Level.* The *Flesch* scores are based on the average number of syllables per word and words per sentence. The *Flesch-Kincaid Grade Level* score rates text based on the U.S. grade-level system, and the *Flesch Reading Ease* score is based on a 100-point scale—the higher the score, the easier the passage is to read.

> You are invited to participate in this research study. The purpose of this form is to give you a written description of the research study and to have you sign this informed written consent. Speaking and singing are sophisticated ways of communication. We are interested in recording samples of your speaking and singing voice during this and subsequent semesters so we can gain a better understanding of the changes in the articulatory, vocal and respiratory systems and effectiveness of vocal training. In order to accomplish this we will ask you to speak and sing. You will stand through the entire experiment. Your speech and singing will be recorded as well as the movements of your rib cage and abdomen, and the activities of respiratory muscles. The respiratory measures will evaluate how far the rib cage and the abdomen move during speaking and singing activities. The activity of your muscles will be recorded using electromyographic techniques to determine which muscles are contracting during your speech and singing. (Mendes, 2000)

The *Flesch-Kincaid Grade Level* for the passage from the Mendes (2000) informed consent form is 12.0—meaning that a 12th-grader should be able to understand the text. What factors should be considered when evaluating the readability of an informed consent form? How could the Mendes (2000) description be made more readable?

In practice, informed consent is traditionally provided to participants in written form with an opportunity for questions and answers. However, some participants require special considerations to insure their understanding of informed consent. For example, special care is needed for participants from different ethnic, cultural, and socioeconomic groups to avoid misunderstandings based on different values and beliefs. Special accommodations are necessary for individuals who are hard-of-hearing, deaf, or blind to insure their comprehension for informed consent.

Researchers have an obligation to openly communicate with participants before, during, and after the study. Before a study begins, individuals should consent to participate or decline to participate based on a full disclosure of information about the study. As a research study progresses, participants should be kept informed and given opportunities to ask questions, express concerns, or withdraw from the study. This is especially important in studies of long duration.

Though full and honest disclosure is the general rule of conduct, *deception* is necessary in planning some experiments. However, deception should only be used in exceptional cases where the truth would make the experiment impossible. For example, an experiment by Collins and Blood (1990) used a "cover story" to disguise the true purpose of their study. The real purpose was to observe nonstutterers' perceptions of stutterers who acknowledged their stuttering and their perceptions of stutterers who did not acknowledge their stuttering. However, participants were informed as follows:

> [Participants were told that] they would be working on a class project examining the effects of working with a stutterer. They were told that they would be working with one of two men and that because their schedules were unpredictable, they would observe videotapes of the two men ahead of time to indicate their preference. They would return a week later to complete the working task with the individual. (Collins & Blood, 1990, p. 77)

After completing the experiment, the true purpose of the experiment and the need for a cover story were explained to participants. If deception is deemed necessary, ethics require that participants are debriefed as soon as possible when a study concludes.

Privacy and Confidentiality

The data collected during the course of a study are *privileged information*. Information gathered about participants is confidential unless otherwise agreed upon beforehand. Data should be used for the present research purpose—not for other purposes. To ensure confidentiality, the anonymity of participants should be established from the start. For example, secret codes can be assigned to participants to protect their true identities. The American Speech-Language-Hearing Association's *Code of Ethics, Principle of Ethics I. (Rules of Ethics K & L)* requires that researchers adequately maintain and appropriately secure research records, and researchers shall not reveal, without authorization, any personal information about research participants (American Speech-Language-Hearing Association, 2003).

Withholding Treatments

Experimental research designs require the random assignment of subjects to two or more conditions. One condition is an experimental treatment, and the other condition is a control condition without treatment. Control groups are also known as comparison groups. A control group is needed to confirm the effect of a treatment on an experimental group. The decision to withhold treatment from persons who may otherwise benefit from the treatment is difficult. However, Hersen and Barlow (1976) challenged the traditional viewpoint that withholding treatment is problematic as follows:

> An oft-cited issue, usually voiced by clinicians, is the ethical problem in withholding treatment from a no-treatment control group. This notion, of course, is based on the assumption that the therapeutic intervention, in fact, works, in which case there would be little need to test it at all. Despite the seeming illogic of this ethical objection, in practice many clinicians and other professional personnel react with distaste at withholding treatment, however inadequate, from a group of clients who are undergoing significant human suffering. (p. 14)

To minimize risk to participants and maximize benefits, researchers should do a risk-benefit analysis when planning their study. Factors such as length of the study and the potential for harm to participants are important considerations. Researchers should weigh potential benefits against potential risks. *Benefit* is a product of the scientific worth of the study and the value to individual participants. *Risk* is any potential harm to the welfare of a participant. For example, if research procedures may cause physical discomfort, emotional stress, or loss of income, these are risks to welfare. However, the possible risks to participants are many and varied as described by Metz and Folkins:

> They might include physical risks from exposure to radiation, electric shock, vocal abuse, and so on. A risk from experimental therapy must be less than the optimal clinical result. There are also emotional risks, such as a potential for embarrassment, invasion of privacy, or undue stress. There may be a risk of adverse financial effects on subjects. There is a risk of misleading subjects (and their families) about their health or abilities. Also, risks which are acceptable with some populations may not be allowed with other groups, such as children. (1985, p. 27)

Special safeguards are needed to protect children, individuals with physical disabilities, students, patients, and other vulnerable populations when they participate in experiments.

Collecting Data, Describing Procedures, and Reporting Results

Before presenting data to the scientific community, a researcher should be certain that observations are accurate. In addition, details of research procedures should be honestly described. A researcher should also describe mishaps that occurred during the course of the study if they might have influenced results. For example, loss of subjects (*attrition*) or breakdown of equipment are significant mishaps and should be reported.

Matters of honesty are addressed in ASHA's *Code of Ethics: Principle of Ethics I. (Rules of Ethics M)* Individuals shall not [. . .] misrepresent services rendered, products dispensed, or research and scholarly activities conducted (American Speech-Language-Hearing Association, 2003). A commitment to honesty is essential for the advancement of science. Dishonesty hinders science and denies the possible benefits to society (cf. Bok, 1999). For example, researchers must replicate experiments in new settings with different participants to confirm results. If the details of studies are not reported accurately and honestly, attempts to replicate results may be fruitless.

When a research study is complete, researchers typically disseminate their results to colleagues by way of professional meetings and scientific journals. In fact, researchers are obliged to share their results with others. If researchers choose not to report publishable results, they are engaging in self-censorship (McGue, 2000). Self-censorship is a disservice to society and the research community because it can have a negative effect on the accumulated record of research. It is important that all publishable research results are made available to colleagues and other interested parties.

Research is often the product of collaboration by two or more investigators. When planning a study, researchers should discuss matters of authorship early to avoid misunderstandings later. Authorship is reserved for those persons who conceive, design, perform, and write a manuscript for publication or presentation. Authorship includes a responsibility for the content of a research report. The first author of a research report is usually the person who contributed most to the study.

Conflicts of Interest in Research

Researchers sometimes face conflicts of interest because of the dual roles that they assume. For example, researchers are often teachers or clinicians, and they move from one role to the other role on a regular basis. As teachers, researchers may unfairly induce students to participate in research. For this reason, teacher-researchers should recruit students from outside their own classrooms. As clinicians, researchers may unfairly recruit patients for their own research endeavors. For this reason, clinician-researchers should recruit research participants from outside their practice or take other precautions to insure that human rights are fully respected.

Honoring Promises and Commitments to Participants

The research investigator should ensure that any and all promises and commitments made to participants are fulfilled. These may include promises such as providing a summary of research results to participants, continuing therapy, or payments for their participation.

Evidence-Based Practice and Ethics in Research

The evolution of research is important to clinical practice because research is the source of evidence for best practices in communication disorders. ASHA's *Code of Ethics: Principle of Ethics I (Rules of Ethics B)* reads: "Individuals shall use every resource, including referral when appropriate, to ensure that high-quality service is provided" (ASHA, 2003). Evaluating research for its application to clinical practice is one of the most important resources available for ensuring that high-quality clinical services are provided. To meet this obligation, clinicians must be able to evaluate the credibility of results and the transferability of research outcomes to their clinical settings.

Scientists prescribe a set of rules and standards to ensure that research is a systematic and ethical endeavor. These rules and standards are collectively known as the *scientific method*. Meline and Paradiso (2003) wrote: "To establish [evidence-based practice], the scientific method must be adopted by clinicians as well as researchers" (p. 274). Herbert, Sherrington, Maher, and Moseley (2001) defined *evidence-based practice* as the systematic use of best evidence typically high quality clinical research to solve clinical problems. Law (2000) proposed eight steps for transferring research results to clinical practice as follows:

1. Clearly identify the clinical problem.
2. Gather information from research studies about the problem.
3. Ensure that you have adequate knowledge to read and critically analyze the research studies.
4. Decide if a research article or review is relevant to the clinical problem.
5. Summarize the information so that it can be easily used in your practice.
6. Define the expected outcomes for the [students, patients, clients, or significant others].
7. Provide education and training to implement the suggested change in practice.
8. Evaluate the practice change and modify (if necessary). (pp. 33–34)

An important consideration when gathering information from research studies (Law's *Step One*) is known as *evidence grading*. Evidence grading is based on the idea that research designs vary in their ability to predict the effectiveness of clinical practices. Higher grades of evidence are more likely to correctly predict outcomes than lower grades of evidence. This hierarchy of research evidence from high to low is graphically depicted in what is known as an *evidence pyramid*.

Figure 2.1 is an example of a research-to-practice evidence pyramid. The pyramid illustrates the evolution of the scientific literature from the base, which begins with an idea, to the top, which ends with an accumulation of research about a specific clinical problem. Moving up the evidence pyramid, the quantity of available literature decreases, but its relevance increases.

The evidence pyramid has two important shortcomings. First, evidence grading considers the general design of studies, but studies of the same general design may differ in quality—some studies are better than others so their outcomes are more meaningful. Second, higher levels of evidence do not exist for all clinical problems. Thus, a specific

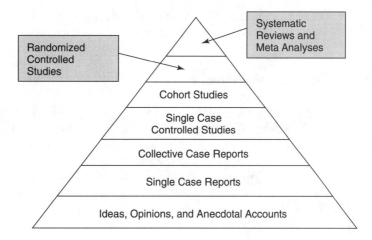

Figure 2.1 A research-to-practice evidence pyramid.

clinical problem—such as how to best manage the language needs of children with Asperger Syndrome—may not be supported by research evidence at the higher levels of the pyramid.

The challenges for clinicians are: (a) to identify the highest level of evidence that is available for answering a specific clinical question, and (b) to evaluate its transferability to the clinical setting. The goal for evaluating research in communication disorders is to provide the knowledge base for accomplishing this task. Where would you expect to find information relevant to each of the seven levels of evidence shown in Figure 2.1?

Conclusion: Ethics in Communication Disorders Research

Research is an honorable endeavor, but disregard for ethics can seriously diminish the effort and may have ill effects on the reputation of science as a legitimate pursuit of the truth. A thoughtful research plan that addresses ethical concerns is paramount, but diligence throughout the research endeavor—beginning to end—is needed to insure that a high standard of ethics is maintained.

CASE STUDIES

Case 2.1 Mrs. Toller's Dilemma

As a speech-language pathologist, your patient, Mrs. Toller, is recruited for an experiment planned by you and Professor Stanford. Mrs. Toller is being treated for swallowing problems. The research plan includes experimental and control groups, and assignment to one or the other group is random. Mrs. Toller has a 50 percent chance of being selected for the experimental (treated) group and a 50 percent chance of being selected for the control (untreated) group. What are the potential ethical issues—and what should you do?

Case 2.2   Authorship for Professor Baker

You are completing a thesis with your advisor, Professor Stangerson. You and Professor Stangerson agreed during the initial planning that you would be the first author and Professor Stangerson would be the second author on any presentation or publications of the results. However, Professor Stangerson received statistical advice from Professor Baker, who is the clinical audiologist, and Professor Stangerson wants to include Professor Baker's name on a presentation of the results. What are the potential ethical issues—and what should you do?

Case 2.3   Deception in the Classroom

You and Professor Gregson are planning a research study in several 4th-grade classrooms to investigate teachers' perceptions of students with speech and hearing impairments. You plan to tell teachers that the study is about nutrition and its effect on classroom behavior. What are the potential issues—and how should you proceed?

Student Exercises

1. In her classic book about lying in public and private life, Sissela Bok examined the reasons why debriefing subjects after deception may not succeed. What does Bok say about deception in experimentation? (Bok, 1999)
2. In 1939, Tudor and Johnson studied 22 children in an Iowa orphanage. The *Tudor Study* received much attention when a report in the *San Jose Mercury News* characterized it as the *Monster Study.* How did Ambrose and Yairi's (2002) report and the *Mercury News* report differ?
3. Informed-consent documents may be difficult to read according to Paasche-Orlow, Taylor, and Brancati's (2003). They gathered research data from templates of informed consent forms at 114 medical schools. *Institutional Review Boards* often post a model (template) for informed consent on their local websites. If your school posts a template for informed consent, what is its readability level?
4. The National Institute on Deafness and Other Communication Disorders (2004) offers guidelines for communicating informed consent to individuals who are deaf or hard-of-hearing. What are their recommendations for facilitating communication with special populations?
5. The National Institutes of Health—Office of Human Subjects Research recommend additional safeguards when research participants have impaired decision-making capacity (Office of Human Subjects Research, 2004). What additional safeguards do they recommend?

CHAPTER

3 Summarizing Observations in Communication Disorders Research

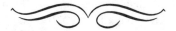

statistics   (stə-tĭs′tĭks) *n.* the collection, organization, and interpretation of numerical data or other values.

Scientists collect data from their observations of physiological and psychological phenomena. Scientific observations become data when they are permanently recorded on paper, magnetic tape, or other media. Data are usually expressed numerically because numbers can be readily organized, analyzed, and interpreted. Assigning numbers to objects or events according to prescribed rules is known as *measurement*. *Statistics* is the branch of science that analyzes and interprets data. The data that scientists collect have different properties depending on their level of measurement. The four levels of measurement are *nominal, ordinal, interval,* and *ratio,* and each is defined by its arithmetic properties.

Levels of Measurement in Communication Disorders Research

The numerical data gathered from observations of physical phenomena and human behaviors must be organized, analyzed, and interpreted to make rational conclusions. The precision of experimental measurements and the choice of statistical tests depend on the properties of the data—and the properties of the data depend on the level of measurement.

Nominal Level of Measurement

The first of four levels of measurement is known as the *nominal level*. Researchers may be interested in categories such as gender or socioeconomic status (low, middle, high) as variables to be studied. These categories are qualitative variables; however, numbers are usually assigned to the categories. The numbers assigned to qualitative variables are referred to as nominal level data or qualitative data. In this case, the numbers are assigned arbitrarily with no numerical meaning. For example, socioeconomic categories may be assigned numbers 1, 2, and 3 (low, middle, high). In this case, arithmetic operations such as [3 > 1] [2 < 4] [4 − 1] and [1 + 3] are not possible. The three remaining levels of measurement—ordinal, interval, and ratio—are concerned with quantitative variables.

Ordinal Level of Measurement

The second of four levels of measurement is known as the *ordinal level*. Ordinal-level data have the property of inequality but lack other arithmetic properties. For example, a rating scale for vocal quality might include the numbers 1, 2, 3, 4, and 5. If 5 is best and 1 is worst, it follows that a rating of 5 is better than a rating of 3, and a rating of 2 is worse than a rating of 4. However, a rating of 4 is not twice as good as 2, nor is a rating of 1 half as good as 2. In other words, ordinal-level data possess the property of inequality but do not have the arithmetic property of equal intervals. As an illustration, equal intervals for a voice rating scale would look like 1_2_3_4_5. However, the true relationship between ratings may be 1_2___3_4__5. That is, the intervals are not necessarily equal. Why are rating scales unlikely to have equal intervals? What steps might you take to insure that the intervals in a 5-point rating scale are nearly equal? How would you design a 5-point rating scale for quality of voice? What "perceptual anchors" would you employ in your design?

Interval Level of Measurement

The third of four levels of measurement is known as the *interval level*. Interval level data possess the arithmetic properties of inequality and equal intervals. Thus, it is appropriate to compute differences but not to multiply or divide interval-level data. For example, the difference between intelligence scores of 100 and 50 equals 50—but it is not appropriate to say that an individual with a score of 100 is twice as intelligent as an individual with a score of 50. Interval-level data have an artificial origin and no *true zero point*. A true zero point indicates the absence of whatever property is being measured. Is it possible to score zero on an intelligence test or a standardized speech-language test or another psychometric instrument? What would zero mean on a standardized achievement test?

Ratio Level of Measurement

A fourth level of measurement is known as the *ratio level*. Ratio-level data have all the properties of interval-level data with the addition of a true zero point that represents total absence of the property. Thus, mathematical operations such as [20 ÷ 10] are possible. Examples of ratio-level data include common measurements such as length, weight, and height. Familiar units of measurement for sound intensity (decibels) and sound velocity (meters per second) are also ratio-level data. What are other examples of ratio-level measurement?

Summary Statistics in Communication Disorders Research

After the dependent variable is measured, researchers must arrange the data in a meaningful way. Such an arrangement of data is called a *data summary*. Data summaries most often appear in *tabular form* (tables). If the total number of observations is small, the individual data can be presented in a *frequency table* such as Table 3.1 adapted from Weaver-Spurlock and Brasseur (1988). Weaver-Spurlock and Brasseur (1988) provided percentages of correct [s] productions for each of three subjects in their research report. Alternatively, the researchers could have presented their data as raw scores—the number of correct productions of [s]. The presentation of data in one form or another depends on the experimenters' preferences.

Data are typically grouped by categories for presentation. Table 3.2 presents grouped data from Abraham and Stoker (1988). Abraham and Stoker (1988) summarized their data within eight categories of manual communication systems. Data presented in tabular form (as displayed in Tables 3.1 and 3.2) are known as *frequency distributions*. Table 3.1 is an example of data organized by participants, and Table 3.2 is an example of data organized by categories. These data could also be presented graphically—such as in line graphs or bar graphs.

Descriptive Statistics in Communication Disorders Research

Frequency distributions are informative; however, shorthand methods for describing the specific features of data are also useful. The most common shorthand methods employed by researchers are known as *descriptive statistics*. A descriptive statistic is a measure of a specific feature or characteristic of a set of data. Descriptive statistics are routinely used to summarize data. Common types of descriptive statistics are: (a) measures of location, (b) measures of variability, and (c) measures of individual location. All are regularly used in communication disorders research.

Table 3.1 Example of data (percent correct on baseline word probes) organized by participants.

	1	2	3	4	5
Participant One	5	8	2	3	—
Participant Two	12	12	7	13	30
Participant Three	0	0	0	2	—

Adapted from Weaver-Spurlock and Brasseur, 1988.

Table 3.2   Example of data organized by categories: Manual systems used by respondents to assess speech and language of hearing-impaired children and youth

	n	Percent
Signed English	73	40.1
ASL	33	18.1
Fingerspelling	31	17.0
Pidgin Sign	23	12.6
SEE II	20	11.0
SEE I	17	9.3
Cued Speech	10	5.5
American Indian	5	2.7

Adapted from Abraham and Stoker, 1988.

Measures of Location

Measures of location are single values that are descriptive of an entire set of data. The value chosen depends on the particular characteristic to be described as well as the measurement level of the dependent variable. Measures of location include two broad categories: (a) central location, and (b) fractiles. Several statistical measures describe central location—the center or middle of a set of data. There are three common measures of central location: (a) mean, (b) median, and (c) mode.

Measurement of the mean requires interval- or ratio-level measurement. The most common measure of central location is the arithmetic *mean* or average. The mean of *n* numbers is their sum divided by *n*. For example:

$$8 + 11 + 15 + 6 + 3 = 43$$
$$n = 5$$
$$mean = 43 / 5 = 8.6$$

The number (*n*) of values in a sample is known as the *sample size*. By convention, the mean is assigned the symbol $\bar{x}$ which is read as *x bar*. The symbol Σ is uppercase *sigma,* the Greek letter for S.

Sigma is the conventional notation for summation. The symbol *x* is assigned to the individual values in a set of data. Thus, the formula for computing the mean is as follows:

$$mean = \frac{\Sigma x}{n}$$

This formula reads as follows: *the mean equals the sum of χs divided by n.* The mean is a valid indicator of central location if the data are normally distributed (or nearly so). If the data include extreme scores at the top or bottom, the mean may be a poor indicator of central location.

Another measure of central location is known as the *median* (mdn). The median for a set of numbers is the midpoint or center of the data. Computing the median requires ordinal-level data or a higher level of measurement. Ranked scores and ratings are common examples of ordinal-level data. If interval or ratio-level data are not normally distributed, the median may be preferred over the mean as a measure of central location.

Computing the median is simple for some sets of data but complicated for others. In all cases, the first step is to arrange the scores in order from low to high. When the sample size is odd and no two values are alike, the median is the middle value. Thus, for the set of data [3, 6, 8, 11, 15], the middle value and the median is 8. When the sample size is even and no two values are alike, the median is the average of the two middle values. Thus, for the set of data [3, 6, 8, 11, 15, 20], the median is [8 + 11 / 2 = 9.5]. Computing the median is more complex when there are data with the same values. For example, the data set [3, 6, 8, 8, 8, 11, 15] contains a three-way tie [8, 8, 8]. However, if the tie is *balanced* (equally distributed) the median is the average of the tied values. Thus, the median for the data set [3, 6, 8, 8, 8, 11, 15] is 8 because the center is balanced with values of 8 on both sides. A second example [3, 6, 8, 8, 11, 15] includes an even number of values with a two-way tie. Because the tie is balanced, the median is the average of the two center values [8 + 8 / 2 = 8].

In the previous example, the median was found by *inspection*. However, unbalanced ties require estimation of the median. For example, a median by inspection is not possible in the data set [2, 4, 5, 5, 5, 7] because the tied value [5] is unbalanced. Therefore, an estimated median is computed in 10 steps as follows:

1. Order the data from low to high.

   2, 4, 5, 5, 5, 7

2. Divide the scores into halves.

   2, 4, 5 | 5, 5, 7

3. Identify an interval ½ unit below and ½ unit above the middle value(s).

   middle value = 5
   interval = 4.5 to 5.5

4. Identify the lower limit (L) of the interval.

   lower limit (L) = 4.5

5. Compute the sample size (n).

   sample size (n) = 6

6. Count the frequency of observations below the lower limit.

   frequency below (Fb) = 2 [2, 4]

7. Count the frequency of observations within the interval.

   frequency within (Fw) = 3 [5, 5, 5]

8. Divide n by 2 (constant) and subtract the frequency below.

   $$(6 / 2) - 2 = 1$$

9. Divide the above value by the frequency within the interval.

$$1 / 3 = 0.33$$

10. Add the value above to the lower limit of the interval.

$$4.5 + 0.33 = 4.88 = \text{est. median}$$

The computations described in steps 1–10 are expressed as a single equation.

$$est.\ median = L + \left[\frac{(n/2) - \Sigma Fb}{\Sigma Fw} \right]$$

The 10 steps are appropriate to estimate the median when using actual observed scores. However, there are situations when data are grouped for analysis. In these cases, the interval is typically greater than one—and special procedures are needed to estimate the median (cf. Hinkle, Wiersma, & Jurs, 1988).

A third measure of central location is known as the *mode*—and it is used exclusively with nominal data. If the researchers' dependent variable consists of numbers assigned to categories with no arithmetic meaning, the mode is the only valid measure of central tendency. The mode is the value that occurs most frequently in the set of data. For example, in the data set [2, 7, 3, 2, 2, 1], the mode is 2. The mode is a relatively uninformative statistic for centrality, but it is the only index of central location for the nominal-level data.

There are two general categories for statistical measures of location in a set of data: (a) measures of central tendency, and (b) fractiles. Statistical procedures are called *fractiles* when they divide a set of data into two or more nearly equal parts. Fractiles identify the proportion of observations above and below them. For example, the median is a fractile that divides data into two equal parts—50% above and 50% below the median. Other fractiles include quartiles, quintiles, deciles, and percentiles. *Quartiles* are statistical boundaries that divide the data into 4 nearly equal parts. They are referred to as the first, second, and third quartiles. The second quartile is also known as the median. *Quintiles* divide the data into 5 nearly equal parts. *Deciles* divide the data into 10 parts, and *percentiles* divide the data into 100 parts. Computing quartiles and other fractiles is similar to computation of the median. The constant [2] in the formula on page 41 is changed according to number of divisions, such as 4 for quartiles, 5 for quintiles, and 100 for percentiles.

Measures of Individual Location

Measures of individual location are used to specify the location of one participant in relationship to a group of participants. They include: (a) ranks, (b) percentile ranks, and (c) standard scores. The simplest procedure—known as *ranks*—orders a group of participants in terms of their performances on some measure from low to high or high to low. For example, in the data set [66, 80, 91, 94, 99], the participant with a score of 94 is ranked second when the scores are ranked from high to low. Another measure of individual location is known as *percentile ranks*. Percentiles are fractiles that divide the data into 100 equal parts. The relative position for an individual within a group of participants is given by the individual's percentile rank. For example, an individual whose score places them at the 80th percentile for the group performed above 80% and below 20% of the group. A third measure of individual location is known as the *standard score*. Standard scores—also known as *z scores*—are raw scores that are converted to standard deviation units. They are useful as indicators of individual location when data are normally distributed. Standard scores are computed from the following formula, where *x* is one participant's score.

$$z = x - mean / standard\ deviation$$

The standard score gives an individual's location relative to the average or mean for the group of participants. For example, if the mean and standard deviation are 100 and 15, respectively, an individual who achieves a score of 130 is two standard scores (*z* scores) above the mean for the group—and an individual who scores 85 is one standard score below the mean for the group. How would you evaluate a score of 115 on a standardized test with a mean of 100 and a standard deviation of 10?

Measures of Variability

Unequal values are a typical trait of the data that is collected in experiments. The degree of dispersion in a set of data is known as *variability* (or spread). The degree of variability is important in research and clinical practice. For example, suppose a child scores 90 on a test that has a mean of 100. The child's score is 10 points below the mean—but what does that mean? Is the child's performance delayed? These questions are answered by knowing the normal variability associated with a test instrument. Measures of central location are not very meaningful without measures of variability. There are many measures of variability including: (a) number of different categories, (b) range, (c) variance, and (d) standard deviation.

Number of Different Categories. Counting numbers of different categories is a simple measure of variability for use with nominal data. For example, if 60% of participants are categorized as low SES, it is useful to know if socioeconomic status is divided into two categories or seven.

Range. Another index of variability is known as the *range*. The range is the largest observed value minus the smallest observed value. In practice, researchers usually report the two extremes, such as "Range is 11–67." The range is helpful when comparing variations between two sets of data. For example, consider the following data:

Sample A: Range = 45 to 90
Sample B: Range = 12 to 99

Sample B appears to be more variable than Sample A. However, knowing the range of scores tells us nothing about the variability of scores falling between the two extremes. An examination of the individual values in Samples A and B ordered from low to high is revealing. The scores in Sample B are fairly distributed from top to bottom. However,

Sample A: 45, 49, 89, 89, 90, 90
Sample B: 12, 22, 49, 65, 79, 99

the scores in Sample A are grouped together at the extremes. Thus, range alone is a poor indicator of variablity. However, the range is the sole measure of variability for *ordinal data*. It is sometimes reported as an indicator of variability for interval and ratio level data, though other measures of variability are more informative.

The Variance.   *Variance* can be calculated for either interval or ratio level data. Variance considers the dispersion of individual values around the mean. Table 3.3 duplicates the values from Samples A and B. In addition, the mean for each sample and the variability of each score in relation to the mean are reported. The differences displayed in Table 3.3 are used for calculating variation in the two samples. The variances are calculated as follows:

1. Square each difference to eliminate plus or minus signs.
2. Sum the squared differences.

$$\text{Sample A} = 2417.34$$
$$\text{Sample B} = 5583.34$$

3. Divide the sum by the number of values minus 1. The number 1 is a constant subtracted from n because the data are a sample of the population. The sample variability is expected to underestimate the population variability—$[n - 1]$ in the denominator compensates for the error in estimation.

$$\text{Sample A} = 2417.34 / (6 - 1) = 483.47$$
$$\text{Sample B} = 5583.34 / (6 - 1) = 1116.67$$

The values computed in step 3 are the variances for Samples A and B. The variance—dispersion of scores around the mean—is greater in Sample B than in Sample A. In other words, individual scores are spread out in Sample B but grouped closer together in Sample A. Variance has a major shortcoming as a descriptive measure because its value is not expressed in the same unit of measurement as the sample scores. For this reason, vari-

Table 3.3   **Example for computation of variances:** Scores and their differences from the mean for samples A and B.

Sample A		Sample B	
Score	**Difference**	**Score**	**Difference**
45	−30.3	12	−42.3
49	−26.3	22	−32.3
89	−13.7	49	−05.3
89	−13.7	65	10.7
90	14.7	79	24.7
90	14.7	99	44.7
Mean = 75.3		Mean = 54.3	

ance is not easily interpreted. However, this fault is overcome by transforming the variance into what is known as a *standard deviation*. The term "standard deviation" was first used in 1893 by Karl Pearson, a founder of the discipline of study known as *statistics*.

Standard Deviation.   The standard deviation *(SD)* is derived from the variation. To express variation in the same unit of measurement as the original data, the square root of the variation is calculated. The square root of the variation in Sample A equals 21.99, and the square root of the variation in Sample B equals 33.42.

$$SD = \sqrt{variation}$$

The standard deviation is easily interpreted. If the *SD* for a set of data is small, it means the values are spread closely around the mean. If the *SD* for a set of data is large, the values are spread further away from the mean.

The Coefficient of Variation.   The coefficient of variation is a measure of relative variation. In some situations, it may be more meaningful to express standard deviation as a percentage of what is being measured. This is particularly true when making comparisons between two or more sets of data. The coefficient of variation (*CV*) is expressed as follows:

$$CV (\%) = (SD / mean) (100)$$

As an example, researchers may want to compare variations in age between two groups of participants with the following characteristics:

Group A: Mean = 30 years, SD = 2.4
Group B: Mean = 26 years, SD = 3.9

$$CV_{GROUP\ A} = (2.4/30)\ (100) = 8\%$$
$$CV_{GROUP\ B} = (3.9/26)\ (100) = 15\%$$

Thus, age is less variable in Group A with a coefficient of variation of 8% versus Group B with a coefficient of variation of 15%.

Statistical Graphics in Communication Disorders Research

The method of *statistical graphics* is defined as "graphical methods for analyzing data" in the classic text by Chambers, Cleveland, Kleiner, and Tukey (1983). The goals of statistical graphics are to: (a) visually communicate information to others, (b) record data compactly, and (c) visually analyze data to learn more about its structure (Chambers et al., 1983). Statistical graphics techniques aim to organize data in ways that facilitate the recognition of patterns in the set of data. They provide information about the distribution and shape of the set of data. For example, statistical graphics techniques display the distribution of data so symmetry and asymmetry are recognizable. Statistical graphics techniques are useful for analyzing data from one variable (univariate data), as well as two variables (bivariate data).

Univariate Statistical Graphics

To examine the characteristics of data from one sample, a variety of statistical graphics techniques are available. The three most common and useful techniques are: (a) histograms, (b) stem-and-leaf plots, and (c) box plots. Histograms are constructed from frequency tables. The intervals chosen for analysis are displayed on the *x*-axis, and the number of scores in each interval is represented by the height of a rectangle. Histograms are like bar graphs except that the columns in bar graphs are separated by a small distance. Histograms are an aid to visualize patterns for quantitative variables, whereas bar graphs are used to graph qualitative variables. Histograms provide information about: (a) central tendency, (b) variability, (c) skewness, (d) presence of outliers, and (e) the presence of multiple modes in the data. Figure 3.1 depicts a histogram and Figure 3.2 depicts a bar graph based on a study of speech-language pathologists' perceptions of their experiences with augmentative/alternative communication (AAC) (Marvin, Montano, Fusco, & Gould, 2003). Figure 3.1 is adapted from Marvin et al.'s (2003) tabled data and represents years of practice for the 71 participants in the study. Figure 3.2 is adapted from a figure in Marvin et al.(2003). It displays the percentages of SLPs recommending AAC across five categories from "almost never" to "daily."

A second statistical graphics technique is known as the *stem-and-leaf display.* Stem-and-leaf displays are analogous to histograms. They provide the same information about the data but in a different way. Figure 3.3 is a stem-and-leaf display for 25 test scores.

The numbers to the left of the vertical lines are *stems* (tens digits), and the numbers to the right of the vertical lines are *leaves* (unit digits). For example, 5 | 2 7 represents the test scores 52 and 57. Like histograms, stem-and-leaf plots display the shape and distribution of a set of data. Another statistical graphics technique is known as the *box plot.*

Box plots—also known as *box-and-whiskers plots*—display the shape and distribution for a set of data with a (a) box, (b) whiskers, and (c) outliers. Figure 3.4 displays the essential features of a box plot.

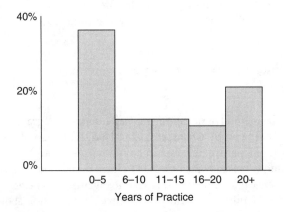

Figure 3.1   A histogram or demographic profile.
Adapted from Marvin et al., 2003.

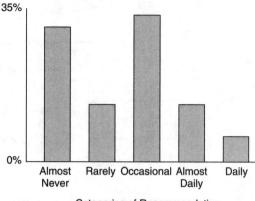

Figure 3.2 A bar graph depicting the percentages of recommendations for AAC.
Adapted from Marvin et al., 2003.

The median is displayed as a horizontal line inside the box. The upper and lower boundaries of the box are the third (Q_3) and first (Q_1) quartiles respectively. The distance between Q_1 and Q_3 is the interquartile range which contains 50% of the data. The whiskers extend from the box to the highest value within the upper limit and the lowest value within the lower limit. Values falling outside the upper or lower limits are designated as *outliers*. Outliers are extreme values that may be misfits in a set of data.

Figure 3.3   Stem-and-leaf display.

```
5 | 2 7
6 | 7 8 9
7 | 1 3 3 5 6 6 7 8 9
8 | 2 3 4 4 5 9
9 | 1 4 5 5 7
```

Technology Note

Though best remembered as a nurse, Florence Nightingale (1820–1910) enlisted tutors to learn mathematics when she was 20 years old. She learned arithmetic, geometry, and algebra years before she became interested in nursing. Florence Nightingale applied her skills with mathematics to medical statistics and invented colorful diagrams to dramatize medical data and to persuade authorities in England to accept her proposals for hospital reform. She is recognized as a pioneer in the graphic presentation of data. Florence Nightingale's work with medical statistics earned her membership in the *Statistical Society of England.*

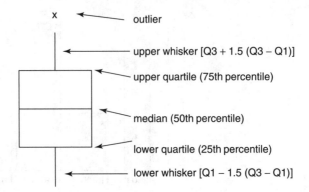

Figure 3.4   Features of the box-and-whiskers plot.

Bivariate Statistical Graphics

Bivariate data consist of the values of two variables, such as height and weight, from one participant. For a group of participants, the values are recorded as (X_1, Y_1) (X_2, Y_2) (X_3, Y_3) and so on. *Scatterplots* are the statistical graphics method of choice for displaying bivariate data. Figure 3.5 is a scatterplot with coordinates labeled X (abscissa) and Y (ordinate). The X coordinate records values for one variable, and the Y coordinate records values for a second variable. Scatterplots display the relationship between two variables in terms of the direction of the relationship (positive or negative) and the shape of the relationship (linear or curvilinear). The scatterplot may also provide evidence of out-

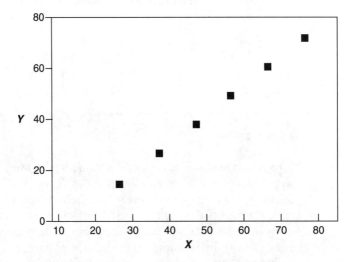

Figure 3.5   Example of a positive and linear relationship between variables X and Y depicted in a scatterplot diagram.

liers or suspicious observations. Figure 3.5 depicts a positive and linear relationship between the *X* and *Y* variables.

Comparing Two or More Samples

Mean plots, standard deviation plots, and box plots can be used to compare the observations from two or more samples. For example, mean plots and standard deviation plots may be used to graph values across time for one participant (time series), or to compare two groups of participants such as experimental versus control groups. Box plots are useful for comparing central tendencies, spreads, and outliers. Figure 3.6 is a comparison between box plots A and B. In what ways do the box plots depicted in Figure 3.6 differ? What other information is available from the box plot comparisons illustrated in Figure 3.6?

Graphing Individual Observations

In addition to statistical summaries for group data, summaries for individual participants may provide additional information. For example, group means may indicate positive increases for a targeted behavior—but individual performances may provide additional information. Figure 3.7 is a graph of clinical outcomes for 10 participants. The outcome is positive for the group as a whole, but an analysis of individual results shows that Participant 2 made no gains and Participant 6 regressed.

Conclusion: Summarizing Observations in Communication Disorders Research

Summarizing observations for presentation in articles and other forums requires the collection, organization, and interpretation of quantitative and qualitative data. To facilitate the handling of data, researchers recognize the inherent differences between nominal, ordinal, interval, and ratio data. The type of data affects the precision and choice of experimental measurements as well as the choice of graphical presentation. A primary goal

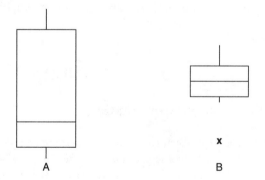

Figure 3.6   A comparison of box plots A and B—with outlier x.

> **Technology Note**
>
> *Microsoft Excel's Tool Menu* includes a *Data Analysis* submenu with histogram and descriptive statistics functions. *Excel's Chart Wizard* includes bar chart, scatterplot, and line graph options—but it lacks a box plot function. Though *Microsoft Excel* does not have a built in box and whisker plot function, researchers can create box plots using stacked bar or column charts and error bars in combination with line or *XY* scatter charts. *Peltier's Excel Page* is a source for *Microsoft Excel Tips and Tricks:* http://peltiertech.com/Excel/index html. Alternatively, researchers can utilize add-ins or macros that supplement *Excel's* usual functions. Data analysis software such as *Minitab* and *SPSS* include many graphics options including box and whisker plots.

for summarizing observations in communication disorders research is to persuade consumers that the researchers' interpretation is the best fit for the data. To this end, a clear and logical presentation of the data in summary and graphical forms meets the objective.

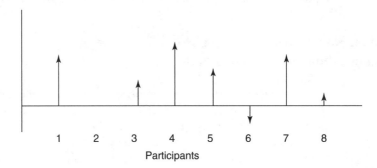

Figure 3.7 A graphic representation of individual participant performances.

CASE STUDIES

Case 3.1   Collaboration and Consultation

Professor Longworth and a research assistant completed a preliminary analysis of data collected from a comparison of two treatment approaches for facilitating language. The average improvement for Group A is 20%, and the average improvement for Group B is 10%. As a consultant, what additional analyses of the data do you suggest to the two researchers?

Case 3.2 Challenge for Clinician-Researchers in Schools

Two clinician-researchers are planning an experiment to test the effectiveness of a new reading fluency program. Because the experiment will be conducted during school hours in 2nd-grade classrooms, the researchers are concerned about possible nuisance variables. What nuisance variables should they anticipate?

Case 3.3 Controlled Experimentation at General Hospital

Researchers at General Hospital collected data from a randomized-controlled experiment where 20 dysphagic patients were divided into two groups. One group received an experimental treatment, and the other group received a placebo treatment. The statistical summaries included the following results:

Experimental Group: mean = 14, SD = 12
Control Group: mean = 8, SD = 2

Based on the preliminary results given, what are your conclusions? Is the experimental treatment an effective one?

Student Exercises

1. Select a research report from a professional journal and answer the following questions. What kinds of data are included? What are the levels of measurement? What summary statistics are reported? What statistical graph methods are used—if none, what methods could have been used?
2. Select a research report from a professional journal. What nuisance variables if any are discussed, and what nuisance variables might they have encountered?
3. What is an acceptable operational definition for an experiment where dysphonic patients are the participants? Write an operational definition for selecting dysphonic participants. Repeat the exercise for cochlear implant patients.
4. For a set of data, the median is 50 and the mean is 50. What do these results indicate?
5. A scatterplot shows a negative and curvilinear distribution for the research team's data set. What do these results indicate?

PART II

Research Designs
for Scientists/Practioners
in Communication Disorders

CHAPTER

4 Group Designs in Communication Disorders Research

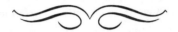

design   (dĭ-zīn′) v. to conceive or fashion in the mind, to formulate a plan, to create or execute in a highly skilled manner.

A research design is a plan that includes protocols for: (a) selecting participants, (b) controlling extraneous variables, (c) implementing treatments, (d) observing variables, and (e) ensuring ethical procedures. Kerlinger (1973) characterized research designs as the blueprints of the research architect and engineer. The value of an experiment depends on the quality of its design. A poor design leads to faulty conclusions, whereas a good design leads to meaningful conclusions. However, a good design alone does not insure the scientific merit of a study.

Formulating hypotheses is a prerequisite to developing sound research designs. A *hypothesis* is a tentative explanation for an observation, phenomenon, or clinical problem that can be investigated. A good design with a poorly conceived hypothesis is unlikely to achieve scientific recognition. The quality of research designs is judged by their ability to answer the research questions and to control extraneous variables. Some research designs are inherently better than others because they are less vulnerable to extraneous variables and various threats to internal validity. A high level of internal validity assures that the relationship between independent and dependent variables can be clearly interpreted. Because weaker designs have poorer mechanisms to control extraneous variables, the risk of reaching faulty conclusions is greater. Though it is important to choose the best research design available, the strongest designs are not appropriate for answering many research questions. According to Kerlinger:

> The most important social scientific and educational research problems do not lend themselves to experimentation although many of them do lend themselves to controlled inquiry of the ex post facto [quasi-experimental] kind. (1973, p. 392)

For this reason, scientists use a variety of research designs. Though there are many different research designs, most designs are variations of a small number of basic designs.

Sampling Designs in Communication Disorders Research

A first step in developing a research design is to identify the population of interest. The *population of interest* or target population consists of all possible individuals who have at least one characteristic in common. For example, the population of adults with aphasia includes every individual who is adult and manifests aphasia. Because the population of aphasics is large and includes many subgroups of aphasia, it may be limited by adding characteristics to the list of characteristics. It is usually not possible to observe every individual in a population—so a sample of individuals is extracted from the target population. A sample is a set of data that represents only a part of the population. The goal for sampling is to extract a relatively small number of observations from a population that will serve as a basis for valid generalizations about the population as a whole.

Sampling Methods

Sampling methods are protocols for gathering a sample from the target population. The sampling method known as *simple random sampling* insures that each individual in the population has an equal chance of being selected for the sample. To carry out simple random sampling, each individual is selected by a chance process, such as drawing numbers from a hat. This kind of random selection is important to insure that results and conclusions can be generalized to the larger target population. Practical constraints dictate that *convenience sampling*—also known as accidental sampling—is sometimes substituted for simple random sampling. The convenience sampling process selects participants from the pool of individuals who are available because of their close geographic proximity or other reasons of convenience. The problem with convenience sampling and other methods that select participants without random sampling is that they severely limit the researchers' ability to generalize results to the larger population.

A viable alternative to simple random sampling of the population as a whole is known as *stratified sampling*. The stratified sampling approach divides the target population into a number of non-overlapping subpopulations (strata), such as geographic regions, and then draws a random sample from each of the subpopulations.

Selecting Participants for Research Studies

Selecting participants for research studies is a critical aspect for all experiments. The characteristics of participants are important considerations for the validity of a study. It is important that researchers establish appropriate selection criteria as a part of their overall plan of study. For example, Gelfand, Schwander, and Silman (1990) adopted a list of 11 selection criteria for their study of normal ears and cochlear-impaired ears. They described their selection criteria as follows:

> [The selection criteria] included (a) measurable auditory thresholds ≤ 110 dB HL (ANSI-1969) at 500, 1000, and 2000 Hz for both ears; (b) no significant changes from prior pure tone thresholds (± 5dB) and speech recognition scores (Raffin & Schafer, 1980); (c) no significant air-bone gaps (Studebaker, 1962); (d) middle ear pressure within ± 50 daPa of atmospheric pressure; (e) static acoustic immittance not exceeding 3000 ohms; (f) no reflex delay (Olsen, Stach, & Kurdziel, 1981); (g) no abnormal threshold adaptation (Olsen & Noffsinger, 1974); (h) no evidence of ear disease; (i) no history or complaints of neurological involvement; (j) normal radiological findings when these tests were done; (k) no evidence of functional overlay; and (l) complaints and history consistent with cochlear involvement. Therefore, the subjects had normal hearing or sensorineural hearing losses attributable to cochlear involvement. (Gelfand et al., 1990, p. 199)

Gelfand and colleagues (1990) supported their choice of selection criteria by referencing authoritative sources. Participant selection criteria should be based on sound principles, and the adoption of established standards is one way to achieve a valid set of criteria. The criteria for participant selection are sometimes discussed (and debated) in professional journals. For example, Logemann (1987) suggested that research participants in studies of dysphagia should be homogeneous for: (a) the nature of the physiologic or anatomic swallowing disorder, (b) the nature of the underlying disease or dysfunction causing dysphagia, and (c) the stage of the disease or recovery process. In similar fashion, Yairi, Watkins, Ambrose, and Paden (2001) discussed their definition of stuttering; Plante (1998) outlined identifying criteria for specific-language impairment; and Leonard and Finneran (2003) reported the effects of grammatical morphemes on mean length of utterance (MLU). Discussions relevant to participant selection issues in communication disorders are found in published sources, including journal articles, research notes, and letters to the editor. Participant selection criteria are important because they affect the internal validity of experiments, the ability to generalize results, and the ability of others to replicate results for confirmation.

The Issue of Representative Samples

Clinical research is most beneficial when participants represent all persons at risk for the behavior or disease being studied. For example, conclusions from samples that only include males limit conclusions to the population of males. In 1990, the National Institutes of Health (NIH) issued a policy statement regarding the inclusion of minorities in clinical research designs and gender composition in clinical studies (U.S. Department of Health and Human Services). In regard to gender composition, the NIH especially encouraged evaluations of gender differences as follows:

> Clinical research findings should be of benefit to all persons at risk of the disease, regardless of gender. [. . .] Public concern requires that clinical studies include both genders in such a way that results are applicable to the general population; exceptions would be those diseases or conditions that occur only in one gender. [. . .] Whenever there are scientific reasons to anticipate differences between men and women with regard to the hypothesis under

investigation, applicants should consider the inclusion of an evaluation of gender differences in the proposed study. (U.S. Department of Health and Human Services, 1990, p. 1)

Since 1990, The National Institutes of Health have updated their guidelines on the inclusion of women and minorities in clinical studies (NIH Office of Extramural Research, 2000).

A representative sample includes individuals from each constituency in the target population, including women and ethnic minorities. If simple random sampling does not produce a representative sample, stratified sampling is an alternative to insure representative samples. In a study of semantic representation and naming in children, McGregor, Newman, Reilly, and Capone (2002) recruited 32 participants in two groups: (a) 16 children with specific language impairment, and (b) 16 typically developing children. They reported the ethnic make-up for both research groups as 70% Caucasian and 30% African-American and Hispanic children. McGregor et al. (2002) noted that the United States population as a whole was made up of 75% Caucasian and 25% minority people. Thus, McGregor et al.'s (2002) sample was a fair representation of the population.

Sample Size and Power

Sample size is the number of participants in a study. Sample size is important because it contributes to the power of a research design. *Power* is the ability of a design to find a treatment effect when one is present. If the power of a design is low, a treatment effect may be hidden. Shadish, Cook, and Campbell (2002) warned that low power is a major cause of false null conclusions in individual research studies.

The power of a design is affected by several factors including: (a) internal validity, (b) measurement reliability, (c) the choice of statistical tests, and (d) sample size. If all else is equal, research designs with more participants will have more power to identify treatment effects and reject the null hypothesis.

Evaluating Selection Procedures in Communication Disorders

An evaluation of an experiment is difficult if participants are not thoroughly described. A detailed description of participants is critical for evaluating the internal validity of an experiment, its ability to generalize conclusions, and the ability to replicate the experiment for confirmation of results. Brookshire (1983) explained the effect of participant descriptions on the evaluation of outcomes as follows:

When an investigator fails to describe adequately the subjects who participated in an experiment, the internal validity of the experiment suffers, because the reader cannot be certain that the observed effects resulted only from the action of the independent variable(s) and not from the action of uncontrolled and unreported subject variables. [. . .] Cursory description of subjects implies cursory consideration of subject characteristics that may have affected the results of the experiment. Careful description of subjects increases the reader's confidence in the believability of the results, and allows the reader to evaluate the outcome of the experiment. (p. 343)

In addition to descriptions of participants as a whole, individual descriptions are important sources of information. Wertz, LaPointe, and Rosenbeck (1984) reflected on past studies that included adults with aphasia as participants:

They [researchers] were careless with individuals within the group. Some patients were sacrificed—their performance submerged in the group mean—to protect, preserve, and promote what we were learning about the disorder. A few conservationists began to report on single cases that questioned the group data. We welcomed both, because without both the future was blank. (p. 51)

Schmitt and Meline (1990) examined 92 research reports with language-impaired children as participants and found that only 30% of the studies included information about individual participants. Regarding the descriptions of adults with aphasia in research studies, LaPointe (1985) noted that people with aphasia are not a homogeneous group, and studies that fail to describe subjects in some detail imply that homogeneity exists.

Yorkston, Smith, and Beukelman (1990) provided individual descriptions for 10 adolescent and adult participants who used alternate and augmentative devices for communication. Their description of individual participants is reproduced in Table 4.1.

A journal may request detailed participant information in their editorial policies. For example, the journal *Aphasiology* advised contributors to include adequate subject description as outlined previously in Brookshire (1983). In addition, the journal *Aphasiology*

Table 4.1   Description of 10 research participants.

Participant	Etiology	Age/Gender	Communication Device	Speech Status
1	CP	13/M	Sharp Memowriter	Some functional
2	CP	30/M	TouchTalker	Some functional
3	CP	21/M	Canon Communicator	Vocalizes as signal
4	TBI	28/F	LightTalker Express	Some functional
5	TBI	18/M	Canon Communicator	Vocalizes as signal
6	CP	27/M	Expanded Keyboard	No vocalization
7	TBI	23/F	Canon Communicator	Vocalizes as signal
8	Aneurysm	30/F	LightTalker Express	No vocalization
9	TBI	22/M	Canon Communicator	Some functional
10	TBI	26/M	Canon Communicator	Some functional

Adapted from Yorkston, Smith, and Beukelman, 1990, Table 1, p. 218.

requested specific participant information for each of 18 variables including age, severity, time since onset, education, handedness, etiology, vision, intelligence, lateralization, mood, gender, and localization.

Single-Group Research Designs in Communication Disorders

A single-group design involves observing one group of participants in two or more conditions. Single-group designs are weak because they lack scientific comparability—a basic requirement for scientific inquiry. In addition, without a comparison group, an important control for extraneous variables is missing. The most common single-group design is the *pretest-posttest design*. Figure 4.1 includes an experimental treatment (X), a pretest observation (O_1), and a posttest observation (O_2). Figure 4.2 is the quasi-experimental (Q) counterpart of Figure 4.1. Figure 4.2 includes a preexisting condition (P), a pretest observation (O_1), and a posttest observation (O_2).

To implement the quasi-experimental design depicted in Figure 4.2, researchers must anticipate the occurrence of the treatment condition P. An alternative is to collect pretest data retrospectively. A retrospective study examines data recorded before the study begins. For example, Shriberg and Kwiatkowski (1987) studied 73 clinical records to discover variables related to the spontaneous generalization of speech. The purpose of studies of this type is usually exploratory. In Shriberg and Kwiatkowski's study, they concluded by suggesting additional variables to be investigated in future studies with the benefit of experimental controls.

Shortcomings in Single-Group Designs

Figures 4.1 and 4.2 have one feature of comparability—participants are compared to themselves. In this way, individual differences are controlled. However, individual comparability alone is too weak to meet the scientific standard of comparability because a large number of extraneous variables remain uncontrolled. The uncontrolled nuisance variables include history factors, maturation factors, multiple-test effects, and statistical regression effects. History and maturation threats are related to the time interval between observations O_1 and O_2. Longer intervals between O_1 and O_2 increase the likelihood that extraneous variables will affect the dependent variable. In addition, because these designs include more than one measurement, test-sensitization and test-practice effects are potential nuisance variables. Finally, if participants have unusually high or low pretest scores, a change in scores may be attributed to a regression effect. The most serious problem with single-group designs is that they provide no means for knowing if extraneous variables have affected the dependent variable. Thus, conclusions based on single-group research designs—especially cause-effect conclusions—should not be viewed as scientifically sound.

Figure 4.1   Single-group pretest-posttest experimental design.

$$O_1 \text{-----------} X \text{----------} O_2$$

Figure 4.2   Single-group pretest-posttest quasi-experimental design. O_1 ---------- P ---------- O_2

Two-Group Research Designs in Communication Disorders

Two-group designs include observations of two groups of participants at different levels of the independent variable. In most cases, one level of the independent variable is a treatment and the other level is a no-treatment (control) condition. The no-treatment condition is an important control for several potential nuisance variables. Because observations of the two groups are made at about the same time, time-related nuisance variables are usually adequately controlled. History and maturation effects should be present in the treatment group and observed as a similar effect in the no-treatment group. In this way, these unwanted effects are of no consequence in the comparison between groups. The potential threats of multiple-test effects and statistical regression are controlled in the same way.

Types of Two-Group Research Designs

There are two basic types of two group designs: (a) independent research designs, and (b) related research designs. Independent designs require the random assignment of participants to experimental and control groups. Figure 4.3 illustrates the basic experimental design with randomization. *Random assignment* means that each participant has an equal chance of being assigned to one group or the other. Random assignment is accomplished by flipping a coin (heads or tails), drawing numbers from a hat, or using a list of random numbers. Randomization reduces the possibility of researcher bias, and— it ensures comparability between the groups.

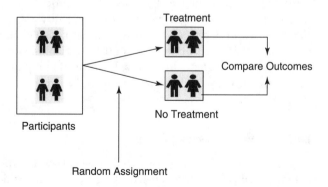

Figure 4.3   A Randomized controlled two-group design.

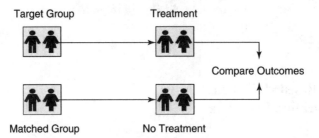

Figure 4.4   A quasi-experimental two-group design.

Figure 4.4 illustrates a basic quasi-experimental design without randomization. Random assignment of participants to groups is not possible in quasi-experimental designs because the independent variable—a classification variable—cannot be manipulated. The quasi-experimental alternative to random assignment is *matching*. Matching procedures attempt to establish group equivalence by matching the two or more groups on the basis of critical variables—variables other than the classification variable. For example, if the classification variable is language status (normal or disordered), critical matching variables might include age, intelligence, and socioeconomic status. The strength of a related two-group design depends on the success of selecting equivalent (matched) groups of participants.

The Issue of Group Equivalence

An important consideration in two-group designs is known as *group equivalence*. Two groups must be equivalent to satisfy the comparability requirement. If the two groups are not equivalent for relevant variables, such as age, gender, and intelligence, conclusions may be meaningless. In the case of independent designs, participants are randomly assigned to groups so the groups should be equivalent. However, in the case of related designs, equivalence depends on matching procedures. To achieve equivalence in quasi-experimental designs, two steps are necessary: (a) identify the relevant variables—those known to be related to the dependent variable, and (b) match the two or more groups of participants on the basis of these variables. For example, if the aim is to compare language-impaired children with a control group of typically developing children, the control group would be matched with the experimental group on the basis of relevant variables such as age and gender.

Basic Two-Group Research Designs

Figure 4.5 is an independent two-group design with an experimental treatment. Its quasi-experimental counterpart (related two-group design) is depicted in Figure 4.6 and includes a preexisting independent variable (*P*) such as a disease or prior clinical diagnosis.

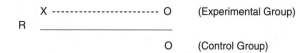

Figure 4.5 Independent two-group experimental design.

Figure 4.5 includes random assignment of participants to groups (*R*)—whereas Figure 4.6 assumes that groups are matched for relevant variables (*M*).

The Figures described in 4.5 and 4.6 are alternatives when pretest observations are not possible. Figure 4.5 exercises control of several potential extraneous variables, so internal validity is relatively high. Figure 4.6 is weaker because it relies on matching procedures to achieve group equivalency, not random assignment. The internal validity of Figure 4.6 is directly related to its ability to match groups on the basis of relevant variables.

Figure 4.7 is a pretest-posttest design with two groups of participants. In addition, the groups are independent because participants are randomly assigned to the two groups. Figure 4.7 adds a pretest so that changes in behavior can be observed. This design has several advantages over other two group designs and is frequently used because it accounts for several extraneous variables. A potential problem with this design is the sensitizing effect of the pretest on participant performances. If the pretest sensitizes participants, external validity is weakened. When test procedures are unusual, difficult, or otherwise likely to affect performance on a subsequent test, pretest-posttest designs should be avoided unless satisfactory precautions can be implemented. Justice, Chow, Capellini, Flanigan, and Colton (2003) adopted the pretest-posttest experimental design illustrated in 4.7, but the research team included two treatments and counterbalanced the order of treatments. This variation of the basic pretest-posttest experimental design is known as an *alternating-treatment design.*

Justice and associates (2003) randomly assigned participants to one of two groups: Group A and Group B. Both groups were given an emergent literacy pretest. Following the pretest, Group A received a 6-week "experimental explicit" intervention program followed by a 6-week "comparison intervention program," and Group B received the 6-week programs in reverse order. Thus, the order of treatments was counterbalanced across subject groups. Both subject groups were posttested at the end of the 12-week intervention period. In addition, "interim" tests were conducted between the two 6-week intervention periods. Thus, the researchers evaluated the overall effects of the two

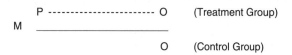

Figure 4.6 Related two-group quasi-experimental design.

$$O_1 \text{ --------- } X \text{ --------- } O_2$$
$$R$$
$$\overline{\qquad\qquad\qquad\qquad\qquad\qquad\qquad}$$
$$O_1 \text{ --------------------- } O_2$$

Figure 4.7 Two-group pretest-posttest independent experimental design.

treatments after 12 weeks, and they evaluated the interim effects of the individual treatments after 6 weeks. Justice et al. (2003) concluded that the "experimental explicit" (name writing, alphabet recitation, phonological awareness) program was superior to the "comparison" (storybook reading) program. Why did Justice et al. (2003) include two intervention programs in their pretest-posttest design? What is an advantage for the alternating-treatment design over the basic pretest-posttest experimental design? What are the disadvantages? The Justice et al. (2003) research team recruited a total of 18 participants for their emergent literacy study. Was the subject sample adequate? What are some possible limitations associated with small subject samples?

Figure 4.8 is the quasi-experimental, related counterpart of the previous design. Like Figure 4.6, the researcher must anticipate the occurrence of the treatment or must collect pretest data retrospectively. Design 4.8 is significantly stronger because it includes a comparison group. However, collected. Potential weaknesses may include problems with group equivalence as well as questionable pretest observations.

Complex Research Designs in Communication Disorders

The complexity of a research design is increased by: (a) adding conditions to the independent variable, (b) adding independent variables, (c) increasing the number of groups, or (d) a combination of a, b, and c. Complex designs are elaborations of basic experimental and quasi-experimental designs.

Multivalent Research Designs

Multivalent designs are complex research designs that include more than two conditions or values of the independent variable. For example, if noise is the independent variable, the research hypothesis may require four or five levels of noise. Figure 4.9 depicts results from a multivalent experiment designed by Cox, Cooper, and McDade (1989). Cox and colleagues used photographs of 10- to 14-year-old females pictured in one of three conditions: (a) wearing a body aid, (b) wearing a post-auricular aid, or (c) unaided. College

$$O_1 \text{ --------- } P \text{ --------- } O_2$$
$$M$$
$$\overline{\qquad\qquad\qquad\qquad\qquad\qquad\qquad}$$
$$O_1 \text{ --------------------- } O_2$$

Figure 4.8 Pretest-posttest two-group related quasi-experimental design.

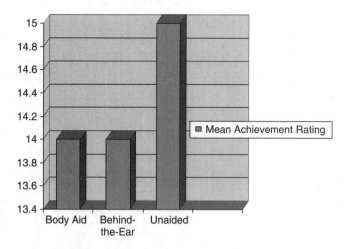

Figure 4.9   Example of a multivalent design.
Adapted from Cox, Cooper, and McDade, 1989.

students who volunteered to be participants rated each photograph on a semantic differential scale. Mean ratings for one of the clusters of attributes—*achievement*—are shown in Figure 4.9. The independent variable—*hearing aid status*—had three conditions: (a) body aid, (b) behind-the-ear aid, and (c) no aid.

Factorial Research Designs

Factorial designs include all possible combinations of the levels of two or more independent variables. In this way, the effects of two or more independent variables are observed within a single study. Factorial designs attempt to model real-life events in which multiple variables may affect behaviors jointly. A combination of two or more variables sometimes produces a change in behavior that is not present when the effects of single independent variables are observed. For example, Mizuko and Reichle (1989) discovered an interaction effect when they examined word categories and graphic symbol systems.

Figure 4.10 is adapted from summary statistics presented in Mizuko and Reichle's (1989) Table 2. Interaction occurred when the observed effect of one independent variable changed as a function of the second independent variable. A picture such as Figure 4.10 provides a graphic representation, which is valuable for interpreting interaction effects. Based on Figure 4.10, the independent variables (symbol system and word category) appear to have interacted in the Mizuko and Reichle (1989) study. In other words, the relationship between nouns, verbs, and descriptors—the three values of the first independent variable—changed substantially as a function of type of symbol system—the second independent variable. An inspection of differences between means at each level

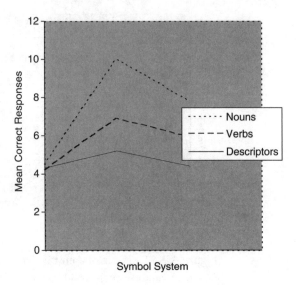

Figure 4.10   Example of an interaction effect.
Data from Mizuko and Reichle, 1989.

of symbol system—Blissymbols, Picsyms, and PCS—suggests the presence of an interaction effect. As an illustration, the difference between nouns and verbs for Picsyms is significantly different from the difference between nouns and verbs for Blissymbols. Thus, an interaction effect is a matter of a difference between differences.

Factorial research designs are generally classified in one of three ways: (a) related designs, in which each participant experiences all treatment conditions; (b) independent designs, in which matched groups of participants experience a single treatment condition; and (c) mixed designs, which combine related and independent variables. Figure 4.11 diagrams a two-by-two factorial design—a basic factorial design with two independent variables and two values for each independent variable. Factorial designs may have additional levels for each variable such as 3 × 5, 2 × 4, and 4 × 5 designs. A factorial design may also include additional independent variables such as 2 × 2 × 2 designs (three independent variables) and 2 × 3 × 4 × 5 designs (four independent variables). The number of possible interactions increases as the number of independent variables increases. Thus, results gathered from factorial research designs become increasingly difficult to interpret as the number of independent variables increases.

Multiple-Group Research Designs

Multiple-group designs include two or more comparison groups along with an experimental or treatment group. Each comparison group typically serves as a control for specific nuisance variables. For example, Figure 4.12 includes one experimental group and two control groups.

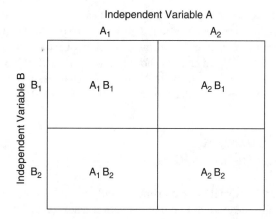

Figure 4.11   Model of a two-by-two factorial research design.

Control Group A controls time-related extraneous variables, such as maturation and history factors, whereas Control Group B controls pretest effects such as test-sensitization and statistical regression. The addition of a second control group in Figure 4.12 manages the shortcomings inherent in pretest-posttest designs. An elaboration of Figure 4.12 is represented by the Solomon four-group design. The Solomon design adds a third control group, which is observed like Group B in Figure 4.12, but does not receive the experimental treatment. The additional comparison group in the Solomon four-group design is intended to control extraneous variable effects that may intrude in the interval between pretest (O_1) and posttest (O_2) observations.

Variations of Three-Group Research Designs

A variation of the three-group design is commonly found in research reports that include specific-language-impaired (SLI) children as participants. Leonard (1979) recommended two comparison groups when studying SLI children—a language-matched control group and an age-matched control group—to yield more meaningful results than permitted with only one comparison group. In a variation of the three-group (two control groups) design, Eadie, Fey, Douglas, and Parsons (2002) recruited 29 children as

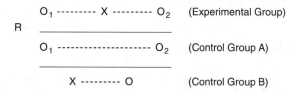

Figure 4.12   Three-group pretest-posttest experimental design.

participants in a study of grammatical morphology and sentence imitation. Their design included two experimental groups—10 specific-language-impaired children and 10 children with Down Syndrome. The control group was made up of 10 typically developing children. What criteria should Eadie et al. (2002) have adopted to insure equivalence between the three groups? What is your evaluation of the research team's sample? What are the factors that affect the power of a research design?

Conclusion: Group Designs in Communication Disorders Research

A wide variety of experiments and research designs exist—and virtually all types of designs are evident in communication disorders. Kerlinger (1973) noted that studying and using research designs is important in order to understand their strengths and weaknesses, as well as their rationale and purpose. Kerlinger's advice is especially meaningful for students of research, prospective researchers, and clinicians who evaluate the extant research literature in communication disorders for evidence-based practice.

CASE STUDIES

Case 4.1   Weak or Strong Design?

Professor Toller and a research assistant plan a pretest-posttest design with one group of participants to test the hypothesis that oral-motor exercises are an effective treatment for speech articulation disorders. As a research consultant, what do you suggest to improve their research design?

Case 4.2   Do Thickened Liquids Work?

Two hospital-based researcher/clinicians are planning a study to determine the effectiveness of thickened liquids for treating oral pharyngeal dysphagia. Their goal is to generalize results to all individuals with dysphagia in the United States. What steps do you recommend for selecting participants?

Case 4.3   Problem of Matching Participants

Two audiologist/researchers are planning a two-group, pretest-posttest quasi-experiment with hearing-impaired children and normal-hearing children as participants. What are the relevant variables that should be considered for matching the two groups of children?

Student Exercises

1. Choose a research report with two or more groups of participants and describe its research design in detail. Why did the researchers include more than one group of participants?

2. Identify the participant selection criteria in one research article in a communication disorders journal. What are the selection criteria, and what is the purpose for including each criteria? What criteria would you have added or deleted from the selection criteria that the researchers specified?

3. Evaluate the selection criteria in a research report that includes a group of at least 20 participants. Given the characteristics of the research sample, what is the population to which the results can be generalized?

4. Identify a factorial research design from a research article in a communication disorders journal. What are the independent variables? Is there evidence of an interaction effect? If there is an interaction effect, how did the researchers interpret the effect?

5. Choose a research report with 20 or more participants. How representative is the sample in relation to the U.S. population? What is the proportion of males and females? Did the study include ethnic groups such as African-Americans, Asian-Americans, and Hispanics? How did the researchers justify excluding particular subgroups in the population?

CHAPTER

5

Qualitative Designs in Communication Disorders Research

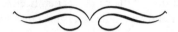

contextual   (kən-têks′ chōō-əl) *adj.* the circumstances in which an event occurs; involving or depending on a context.

Qualitative research refers to a family of more than 30 approaches and designs. It has its origins in the field research of anthropologists as they observed the day-to-day lives of their subjects. Qualitative research has a long history in the social sciences, and its use is on the rise in communication disorders. The contemporary interest in qualitative research—an alternative to quantitative research—has stimulated topical papers, presentations, and qualitative studies in communication disorders, as well as special interest groups devoted to qualitative research. The *Qualitative Interest Group* at the University of Georgia (2004) characterized qualitative research as a general approach to scientific inquiry and more as follows:

> The label "qualitative research" is used generically for approaches to inquiry that depend on elaborated accounts of what we see, hear, taste, touch, smell, and experience. It has roots in cultural anthropology, field sociology, and the professional fields. Qualitative research includes field research, case study research, ethnography, document and content analysis, interview and observational research, community study, and life history and biographical studies. Other names sometimes used as synonyms for qualitative research are interpretive, naturalistic, phenomenological, and descriptive. Qualitative research is associated with such theories as symbolic interactionism, constructivism, and ethnomethodology. Qualitative researchers have a lot of fun, which sustains them through the aggravation, frustration, uncertainty, and sheer slipperiness of most of the approaches to inquiry considered qualitative. (*Qualitative Interest Group*, 2004)

In contrast to quantitative methods, *qualitative research* depends largely on descriptions, categories, and words, whereas quantitative research depends largely on numbers and statistics. Qualitative research designs typically include seven steps. Qualitative researchers do the following:

1. Observe events or ask questions with open-ended answers.
2. Record what is observed, said, or done.
3. Interpret the data.
4. Return to further observe or ask more questions.
5. Repeat steps 2–4 (*iteration*).
6. Develop formal theories to explain the data.
7. Formulate conclusions and generate hypotheses.

Qualitative data are usually detailed, in-depth descriptions of the phenomena being studied. The data are derived from a variety of sources including field notes, clinical records, audio- and videotape transcriptions, photographs, and any other source that lends itself to understanding the phenomenon through firsthand experience. The purpose of qualitative research is to describe, explore, or generate ideas, thoughts, and feelings and to form hypotheses that can be tested by quantitative research designs. The *qualitative research approach* excels at understanding individual differences and similarities, whereas quantitative research excels at understanding group similarities and differences. The qualitative research approach is characterized by ten interrelated themes or assumptions (Patten, 2004). The ten themes are as follows:

1. *Naturalistic inquiry:* Qualitative research focuses on persons, topics, locations, or events in their natural setting such as classrooms, homes, neighborhoods, or cultural milieus.
2. *Inductive analysis:* Qualitative researchers begin with specific examples or facts, formulate questions, and end with general principles or theories.
3. *Holistic perspective:* Qualitative researchers assume that the whole is greater than the sum of its parts. Whatever the focus of inquiry, each action, communication, or other aspect of the milieu is viewed as a part of the whole. The parts are dependent on one another and interrelated.
4. *Thick description:* Qualitative researchers gather detailed information about the phenomenon of interest, and they typically "triangulate" data from multiple sources such as field notes, in-depth interviews, audiotapes, and other sources.
5. *Personal contact and insight:* Because qualitative research requires direct experience with the phenomenon of interest, personal biases are unavoidable. Qualitative researchers are aware of personal biases, acknowledge them throughout the course of the study, and temper their influence.
6. *Dynamic systems:* Qualitative research is a dynamic process wherein answers, questions, and theories are subject to change throughout the course of the study.
7. *Unique case orientation:* Qualitative researchers assume that each case is unique and therefore deserves detailed and in-depth study.
8. *Context sensitivity:* Qualitative researchers appreciate the contextual variables that influence the phenomenon of interest, whether the topic of interest is a person, place, location, or other phenomena.
9. *Empathic neutrality:* Qualitative researchers are nonjudgmental and remain neutral observers throughout the course of the study.
10. *Design flexibility:* Qualitative researchers redirect their focus, generate new questions, and research other topics as they emerge during the course of a study.

Qualitative research is an alternative to quantitative methods when individual perspectives are more important than group generalizations, and when the primary purpose is exploratory or to generate theories as opposed to testing hypotheses. According to Green and Britten (1998), the individual observations that characterize qualitative research are credible evidence for clinical practice. Green and Britten remarked as follows:

> Clinical experience, based on personal observation, reflection, and judgment, is also needed to translate scientific results into treatment of individual patients. Personal experience is often characterized as being anecdotal, ungeneralisable, and a poor basis for making scientific decisions. However, it is often a more powerful persuader than scientific publication in changing practice. (1998, p. 1230)

Clearly, qualitative research is a viable approach to scientific inquiry in communication disorders, and it has important implications for research to practice issues.

Foundations of Qualitative Research

The general approaches to qualitative research include: (a) ethnography, (b) phenomenology, (c) field research, and (d) grounded theory. The major qualitative approaches are general ways of thinking about conducting qualitative research. Each approach typically specifies: (a) the role of the researcher, (b) the stages of the research process, and (c) the methods of data analysis (Trochim, 2004). However, the various approaches may overlap, combine, and otherwise blend so that distinctions between the various approaches are blurred. The first of the several general approaches to qualitative research is known as ethnography.

Ethnography

The *ethnographic approach* has its roots in anthropology. *Anthropology* is the social science that studies the origins and social relationships of human beings. One of the most famous anthropologists was Margaret Mead whose detailed descriptions of child development and adolescent behaviors in the Manus and Samoan cultures helped define the ethnographic approach. Ethnographers typically focus on an entire culture of people. The definition of *culture* was once limited to geographic location and ethnicity, but it has broadened to refer to any group or organization including clinical groups, schools, classrooms, and businesses. The most common ethnographic method is *participant observation,* wherein the researcher is immersed in the culture and becomes an active participant. Researchers assume *outsider* or *insider* perspectives, depending on their qualifications. For example, an ethnographer who studies the culture of medical speech-language pathologists with no speech-language pathology training is an *outsider* and assumes an outsider's perspective. An ethnographer who conducts the same study with speech-language pathology credentials is an *insider* and assumes an insider's perspective.

Damico and Simmons-Mackie (2003) described the primary characteristic of ethnographic study as flexible in the various approaches that can be applied to data collection. Ethnographic researchers typically adopt many different methods for gathering data, including in-depth interviews, focus groups, document analysis, audio- and videotape analysis, introspection, and lamination. For example, Stillman, Snow, and Warren (1999) collected data from individual interviews, small group discussions (focus groups), and videotapes of speech-language pathology students interacting with pervasive developmental disordered (PDD) children.

Data are verified and conclusions are strengthened by combining data-gathering methods in the process known as *triangulation*. Triangulation of data involves comparing and contrasting data that are collected at different times, by different methods, and in different locations. Another technique for verifying data is referred to as *lamination*. Damico and Simmons-Mackie described lamination as follows:

> When employing lamination, the researcher analyzes the collected data and forms tentative conclusions. Once this is done, the conclusions are verified through a different type of cross-comparison process; the researcher may ask the participants in the ethnography what they believe was happening when certain communicative or learning behaviors were observed. In this way, the researcher adds another layer of interpretation to the data so that the actual results or findings can be cross-referenced. In a sense, the term "lamination" is a metaphor for layering on different levels of interpretation. (2003, p. 137)

The ethnographic approach to qualitative research has no preset limits as to what will be observed, and it has no prescribed ending point. Rather, the researcher determines when the study will conclude. Damico and Simmons-Mackie (2003) described ethnography as a promising approach to qualitative research for communication disorders, inasmuch as it is particularly well-suited for investigating complex social and cultural phenomena such as diversity, development, classroom performance, rehabilitation, and service delivery. Another general approach or way of thinking about qualitative research is known as phenomenology.

Phenomenology

Phenomenology is a school of thought that focuses on individuals' experiences, perspectives, and their unique interpretations of the world. The phenomenologist seeks to understand how the world appears to others. Phenomenology is more a philosophical understanding of the world than a methodological approach to qualitative research. Phenomenologists typically reject speculation and the acceptance of unobservable phenomena, oppose the notion of *naturalism* (a metaphysical theory which holds that all phenomena can be explained mechanistically in terms of natural causes and laws), and phenomenologists believe that only objects in the natural world can be known. As an interpretative practice, phenomenology is a unique approach to qualitative research.

Cream, Onslow, Packman, and Llewellyn (2003) adopted the phenomenology approach to study experiences after therapy with prolonged speech techniques of people who stutter. *Prolonged speech* is the term applied to the speech patterns that result from therapies characterized as "smooth speech," "easy speech," and "precision fluency shaping" (Cream et al., 2003). The Cream et al. research team described their methodology as follows:

> Phenomenology is characterized by the focus on phenomena as immediately experienced. The methodology as described by Van Manen (1990) was applied to this study, because

none of the authors stutter, and could experience speech after PS (prolonged-speech] therapy directly. This approach incorporates other people's experiences and their reflections of their experiences were 'borrowed' (Van Manen, 1990: 62) for the purpose of the investigation. The investigator aimed to assist participants to focus on the immediate experience on which they were reflecting, rather than on their accepted customary ways of interpretation. These verbal descriptions of experiences were transcribed into texts that provided data for the analysis. (2003, p. 382)

Another general approach or way of thinking about qualitative research is known as field research.

Field Research

Field research is a broad approach to qualitative research that is characterized by observations of phenomena in their natural state or context. Field researchers typically collect detailed notes that are subsequently categorized and analyzed in a variety of ways. Field research is integral to the ethnographic approach to qualitative research. As such, the field research approach is well represented in communication disorders research, such as Bloom's (1970) classic study of children's early language development. Bloom collected tape-recorded conversations from several young children in naturalistic situations— during eating, dressing, toileting activities, and during play with a peer. Another general approach to qualitative research is known as grounded theory.

Grounded Theory

The grounded theory approach to qualitative research aims to develop theories about the phenomena of interest that are firmly grounded in observation. Overall, grounded theory prescribes a complex, iterative process of observation and verification. According to Damico and Simmons-Mackie (2003), *grounded theory* was proposed to accomplish three analytical strategies. They described the three strategies as follows:

> First, the researcher should periodically step back and ask, "What's going on here? and "Does what I think here fit the reality of the data?" Second, researchers should maintain an attitude of skepticism so that all information from any source is provisional in nature until it is checked out by "playing it against the data." [Third], in order to make best use of theoretical sensitivity, the researcher should follow specific procedures unique to qualitative research and its purposes. (Damico & Simmons-Mackie, 2003, p. 138)

Grounded theory does not prescribe a specific ending point for the study. Rather, the process of observation, verification, and iteration continues until the researcher is satisfied that the data are sufficient to develop a credible theory about the phenomenon of interest. There are few examples of the grounded theory approach in the communication disorders literature. However, Damico and Simmons-Mackie (2003) characterized grounded theory as a promising approach for effectively analyzing phenomena in communication disorders. An example of research rooted in grounded theory is Reid, Hertzog, and Snyder's (1996) study. They described their rationale, method, and research question as follows:

Finally, in looking at how a system functions, we need to consider process as well as outcomes. Therefore, a study was undertaken to explore and describe the perceptions of parents and ADHD about their experiences with the school system. Grounded theory methods were used to develop a tentative model of the process and to suggest hypotheses concerning factors likely to influence the course of the process. Our investigation asked the question: "How do parents perceive the process they have gone through in obtaining services for their children with ADHD?" (Reid et al., 1996, p. 74)

Qualitative Research Designs and Methods

Six common qualitative research designs are: (a) the case study, (b) discourse analysis, (c) kinesic analysis, (d) direct observation, (e) participant observation, and (f) the unstructured in-depth interview. Each of the six qualitative research designs is distinguished by its methods for data collection and its methods for analysis. One of the most common designs for collecting qualitative data is the *case study method.*

The Case Study Method

A case study is an intensive observation of a person, topic, location, or event. Damico and Simmons-Mackie (2003) identified three types of case studies: (a) *intrinsic case studies* seek to gather specific information about a person, place, or thing in a particular context, (b) *instrumental case studies* seek to better understand an issue, generate a theory, develop or modify an existing theory, and (c) *collective case studies* seek to investigate a general phenomenon by way of combining several cases. The qualitative case study method has a long tradition in the social sciences, psychology, education, communication disorders, and other disciplines. Freud used the case study method to develop his theory of psychoanalysis, and Piaget used the case study method to develop a theory of cognitive development. Their observations were qualitative in nature, but many case studies are based on quantitative data. For example, Sapir, Spielman, Ramig, Hinds, Countryman, Fox, and Story (2003) studied the effects of an intensive voice treatment on one person, and their data were quantitative. In contrast, DePaul and Kent (2000) collected qualitative data in their case study which focused on speech intelligibility. DePaul and Kent (2000) described their case study as follows:

> This study describes the effects of listener proficiency and familiarization on judgments of speech intelligibility and speech severity associated with a progressive dysarthria. Speech performance was followed longitudinally for 39 months postdiagnosis for a man with ALS. The subject's spouse served as a highly familiar listener whose speech severity and intelligibility were compared to those of 24 unfamiliar listener-judges. (p. 230)

Several questions arise from Depaul and Kent's (2000) explanation. Who were the participants in the DePaul and Kent (2000) case study? Was the primary focus of their study a person, a place, or a topic? DePaul and Kent (2000) concluded that their results suggest speech-language pathologists should include listener training in their standards of practice for dysarthria treatment.

Another example of qualitative research is a case study reported by Strum and Nelson (1997). They described their study as follows:

> A multiple-case design was used to investigate the discourse of formal lessons in five class-rooms at each of the grade levels—first, third, and fifth. The 15 participating classrooms were chosen to offer a "typical case" perspective on general education elementary classrooms (Bogdan & Biklen, 1992), without implying that they represent all elementary school class-rooms. (Strum & Nelson, 1997, p. 256)

Strum and Nelson (1997) selected 15 classrooms (locations) as the focus of their case study. Their study qualifies as a collective case study because it combines studies of several (15) different classrooms. Why did Strum and Nelson adopt the collective case study method?

The goal of Strum and Nelson's (1997) qualitative analysis was as follows: "[to] reduce the data across the multiple cases (classrooms) to patterns, categories, and themes, and to interpret the information that emerged into a larger consolidated picture" (p. 257). To that end, they identified 10 formal discourse rules such as: "Teachers mostly talk and students mostly listen—except when teachers grant permission to talk." Based on their analyses, Strum and Nelson (1997) concluded that discourse and social interaction level rules play a role in helping students know what to say, when to say it, and how to say it in whole-group discussions. Furthermore, they suggested that speech-language pathologists might collaborate with classroom teachers when a student has a problem understanding discourse rules.

Overall, the case study method has a lengthy history of contributions to communication disorders in regard to generating theories and generating clinical practice ideas. The case study method is a flexible design which can focus on clinical cases, geographic

---

Technology Note

According to Gibbs, Friese, and Mangabeira (2002), the tape recorder is an early example of technology in qualitative research. Today's digital audio and video technologies allow data to be analyzed with the help of powerful computer software tools. These applications are collectively known as computer assisted qualitative data analysis (CAQDAS) tools. Software applications for analyzing text include *Systematic Analysis of Language Transcripts (SALT)* (Language Analysis Lab, 2003) and *Computerized Profiling* (Long, 2003). Word processing applications such as MS Word and WordPerfect have text analysis capabilities, but more powerful text analysis engines are incorporated in QDA Miner, WordStat, Open Text, Collate, TACT, and WordCruncher—examples of the many QDA programs available. A comprehensive list of QDA resources is included in the web pages of *http://qualitativeresearch.uga.edu*. Digital technology is a boon to many qualitative researchers, but others criticize its use (cf. Gibbs et al., 2002). What do you see as possible advantages and disadvantages for CAQDAS?

locations, specific topics, or particular events. It is an especially effective method for scientific inquiry when it is combined with quantitative methods or other qualitative designs.

The Discourse Analysis Method

Discourse analysis is concerned with language use (spoken or written) beyond the boundaries of an utterance or sentence. For example, early literacy instruction was the focus of a study reported by Culatta, Kovarsky, Theadore, Franklin, and Timler (2003). Their purpose was to evaluate the effectiveness of language and literacy instruction with 31 children from Head Start classrooms. Culatta and colleagues combined aspects of the ethnographic approach with conversational analysis—a component of the discourse analysis method. Culatta et al. (2003) explained as follows:

> This investigation drew upon two approaches to studying language as social interaction: the ethnography of communication and conversational analysis. Borrowing from the ethnography of communication, rhyming activities were analyzed as speech events; borrowing from conversation analysis, the instructional interactions were examined on a conversation turn by conversational turn basis. (p. 177)

Damico and Simmons-Mackie (2003) cited numerous examples of conversational analysis in the aphasia research literature. For example, Oelschlaeger and Damico (2000) applied the conversational analysis method to study a conversational partner's strategies when assisting with the word searches of an aphasic partner. The researchers described their design as follows:

> The analytic objective of conversation analysis is examination of a focal conversational event to discover how it is systematically organized and accomplished by participants (Levinson, 1983). The basic analytic tool is a rich descriptive analysis of conversation sequences and the turns at talk within the sequences with findings inductively derived from these behavioral observations (Levinson, 1983). As in all varieties of qualitative research, extensive data collection, detailed description of the data collected, and various ways of comparing and contrasting these data serve to verify any findings. (Oelschaeger & Damico, 2000, p. 208)

Clearly, discourse analysis methods have many applications in communication disorders research, including the exploration of conversational strategies with typically developing children and adults and those with disorders. Oelschlaeger and Damico (2000) summarized the importance of the investigation of partner strategies in the final paragraph of their report as follows:

> The clinical contribution of this study (combined with Oelschlaeger's [1999] report) is the explication of how participatory word search strategies are accomplished in natural conversation. Clinicians should be able to use this information to determine whether conversational partners are using and capitalizing on strategies or may benefit from explicit training of strategies. (p. 219)

Given Oelschlaeger and Damico's concluding remarks, what are the options for continuing this line of research? Is there a role for hypothesis testing in regard to training conversational strategies?

The Kinesic Analysis Method

Kinesiology is the study of communication through body movements, facial expressions, and gestures. *Kinesic analysis* examines what is communicated through these nonverbal movements, postures, and gestures. Kinesic analysis is usually combined with other qualitative methods such as discourse analysis in order to triangulate the data. The qualitative data collected in kinesic studies are usually systematically arranged in categories. For example, Ekman and Friesen (1969) classified nonverbal communications into five categories. The five categories include the following:

1. *Emblems* are nonverbal messages that have a verbal counterpart. The "OK sign" is an example of a hand gesture that has the verbal counterpart *okay*.
2. *Illustrators* are nonverbal body movements and gestures that do not have a clear verbal counterpart. They are usually used to illustrate what is being said.
3. *Affective displays* are body movements or facial expressions that communicate certain affective states or emotions. They are often used less consciously as illustrators.
4. *Regulators* are nonverbal signs that replace, modulate, and maintain the flow of speech during a conversation. Examples of regulators include nods of the head and eye movements.
5. *Adaptors* include postural changes and other body movements that are carried out at a low level of awareness. Examples of adaptors include sitting postures and general body orientation. Adaptors are easily misinterpreted. They are sometimes thought to be indicators of private thoughts. On the other hand, they are frequently used to resolve a specific physical situation such as to achieve a more relaxed seating position.

Kinesics is an important part of communication, but body movements and facial expressions can be easily misinterpreted. Therefore, the analysis of kinesic data is often difficult, and credibility is sometimes questionable. Kinesics is also known to be culturally bound, so the potential for misunderstanding body movements and gestures increases across cultural boundaries. Another method for qualitative analysis is known as *direct observation*.

The Direct Observation Method

The direct observation method entails detailed and systematic observations of a person, location, event, or topic of interest without the researcher's intrusion or participation in the scene. In this way, researcher biases are minimized. The direct observation method utilizes many techniques for collecting data including note taking, video- and audio-recordings, and photographs. Typically, data collection is triangulated from different sources to insure the credibility of observations. Direct observation was the principle method employed by Piaget in his classic studies of infant behavior and cognitive development. Wadsworth (1989) offered the following description of Piaget's work in the context of the era in which Piaget lived:

> In America, experimental research in psychology typically concerned itself with hypothesis testing, rigorous control of experimental variables, and treatment of data with sophisti-

cated statistical procedures. Most of Piaget's research was not experimental in these ways. He did not typically employ elaborate statistics to test hypotheses or use control groups in his research. From his work in Paris in Binet's clinic, Piaget evolved a clinical-descriptive technique that became a trademark for his work. It essentially involved asking individual children carefully selected questions and noting their responses and their reasoning for those responses. In other cases, data were no more than the observation of infant behavior. It was difficult for American Psychologists to consider these techniques experimental because Piaget's methodology bore little resemblance to American experimental psychology. Piaget's work was basically observational, though it was invariably systematic and his analyses were exceedingly detailed; they were designed to detect developmental changes in cognitive functioning. (pp. 5–6)

A contemporary example of the direct observation method and its application is described in a report by Ukrainetz and Fresquez (2003). Ukrainetz and Fresquez employed multiple data sources including open-ended interviews, written reports (historical data), and direct observations with field notes. The direct observation phase of their study was characterized as follows:

> One observation, with field notes, of 30–60 minutes, of each teacher her class, and several observations of each SLP carrying out therapy. The SLP observations took place wherever therapy was occurring: speech room, resource room, or classroom. The first author transcribed the field notes, expanding and clarifying from the handwritten work within 2 days of taking the notes. (Ukrainetz & Fresquez, 2003, p. 287)

In this case, one of the researchers took field notes and reviewed them within two days of the direct observation. What, if any, steps would you suggest to improve the credibility of the researchers' procedures for direct observation?

The direct observation method assumes that the researcher will remain somewhat detached from the scene. To this end, modern technology allows remote observations via one-way mirrors and video cameras.

The Participant Observation Method

In contrast to direct observation, the participant observation method requires the researcher to become a participant in the culture or context that is being observed. The *participant observation method* is more demanding than direct observation because the researcher must acclimate to the situation and become an accepted member in the scene. A classic example of the participant observation method is Bloom's (1970) detailed account of her observations of young children acquiring language. Bloom's account is as follows:

> With a few brief exceptions, the investigator, who was well known to the children, was present in the observation sessions and interacted freely with the child. The mothers were present less than one-third of the time and the fathers only occasionally. The investigator's participation was necessary for noting features of behavior and environment in order to transcribe the tape recordings subsequently, and for maintaining the relative uniformity of the sessions for the three children. The samples were less than "naturalistic" to this extent. (1970, p. 16)

Bloom suggested that the observations that were accomplished in the children's homes may have been less than natural because of her presence. The researcher's observations began when the children were between 19 and 21 months of age. What is your evaluation of the effect of Bloom's presence on the observations that were recorded? Did Bloom's presence have a significant effect?

The participant observation method typically demands more time and resources than direct observation because of the need to immerse oneself into the context of the study. Thus, there are relatively few examples of the participant observation method in the communication disorders literature. Nonetheless, the participant observation method is a powerful method for observing cultural variables, language development, and other social behaviors from an *insider's* perspective.

The Unstructured In-Depth Interviewing Method

The unstructured interview is a widely used method in qualitative research circles for gathering data. The method is characterized by open-ended questions, no formal structure, and an iterative process of questions, answers, and generating more questions based on previous answers. Whereas *structured interviews* focus on answers to a narrowly defined set of questions, *unstructured interviews* focus on broad topics and concepts. The unstructured interviewing method is especially well-suited to exploring sensitive, emotional, and personal issues. Unstructured interviews can be conducted with individuals or groups of participants. Marketing researchers use *focus groups*—individuals with characteristics matching their consumers—to evaluate products that are in various stages of development. In this way, the researchers seek to assess user needs, feelings, and preferences before a product is launched. Focus group sessions are typically free-flowing and relatively unstructured, but the moderator must follow a preplanned script of specific issues and establish goals for the type of information to be gathered. Online forum discussions and newsgroups are sometimes used to approximate focus groups; however, at least two disadvantages are apparent: (a) Internet users may present an unwanted bias because of their unique attributes, and (b) confidentiality of online data is problematic. Stillman, Snow, and Warren (1999) employed focus groups (small group discussions) in combination with individual interviews as means to gather data in their investigation of encounters between speech-language pathology students and children with Pervasive Developmental Disorder (PDD).

The use of *unstructured in-depth interviews* is relatively common in the communication disorders literature. One such example is a qualitative study that was reported by Ukrainetz and Fresquez (2003). They gathered data from multiple sources (open-ended interviews, direct observations, and student files) to examine how speech-language pathologists carried out their roles in schools. Ukrainetz and Fresquez (2003) described their interview protocol as follows:

> Audiotaped open-ended interviews with each SLP and teacher participant, transcribed by the second author and two research assistants, and a few clarifying questions by e-mail to the SLPs following the data collection periods. Topics included the following: education and work history; degree to which educational programs and practices were mandated; caseload, service structure, and assessment methods; teaching practices; explaining the terms *language* and *phonemic awareness*; role in reading and writing instructions; and roles and interconnections of the remedial educators. (p. 286)

The two researchers, Ukrainetz and Fresquez (2003), utilized email as a follow-up to their face-to-face interviews of speech-language pathologists. Meline and Mata-Pistokache (2003) considered advantages and disadvantages related to the use of email in professional practices. In the context of the Ukrainetz and Fresquez (2003) study, what are advantages and disadvantages for using email in research?

Mastergeorge (1999) adopted an unstructured interview as the method of data collection in a study designed to "explore families" use of metaphoric language and its role as a mediator in revealing family members' perceptions of diagnosis and disorder" (p. 246). Mastergeorge (1999) described the interview procedure as follows:

> Family stories were collected about their experiences in coping with disabilities. Each family was interviewed twice, with each interview lasting approximately 3 to 4 hours. When possible, the families were interviewed in the privacy of their own homes by graduate students trained in ethnographic interviewing techniques. (pp. 247–248)

Mastergeorge reported that interviews were conducted in the families' homes when possible. How might the environment in which an interview is conducted affect the data? Based on the data that she collected from open-ended interviews, Mastergeorge (1999) concluded that metaphor is a powerful vehicle that families use to voice their experiences.

Credibility and Transferability in Qualitative Research

Lincoln and Guba (1985) proposed *credibility* and *transferability* as two criteria for evaluating qualitative research. Credibility is the criterion used for evaluating the believability of results. Qualitative research endeavors to understand phenomena from the participants' perspectives. A study's results and conclusions are credible inasmuch as they accurately reflect the participants' feelings, opinions, intentions, and actions. Credibility is improved by employing multiple methods and triangulating data from different sources. Five techniques for evaluating credibility are:

1. *Integrity of the observations.* Factors to consider are the length and persistence of observations and the presence of triangulation of data by multiple sources.
2. *Peer debriefing.* Factors to consider are the use of a devil's advocate perspective and the use of disinterested parties to assess conclusions.
3. *Negative case analysis.* Factors to consider are revision of conclusions to account for known cases and recasting conclusions until they fit observed reality.
4. *Referential adequacy.* Factors to consider are unanalyzed data set aside and analyzed after conclusions are drawn to see if they match.
5. *Member checks.* Factors to consider are the sharing of conclusions with the participants and assessing the match between researchers' conclusions and the participants' reality.

The credibility of qualitative research is a basic requirement for its acceptance; however, transferability of the results and conclusions is also important—especially for clinical practice. *Transferability* refers to the extent that results can be transferred from a study to other persons, locations, events, or other contexts. The transferability of qualitative research results is improved by detailed descriptions of research methods and thorough descriptions of the focus and context of studies. The ability to successfully transfer results to a person or location is determined by the consumer's evaluation. Thus, speech-language pathologists are responsible for evaluating the transferability of qualitative research results to their clinical practices, and audiologists are responsible for evaluating the transferability of results to their practices. The consumers (teachers, audiologists, and SLPs) evaluate the consistency of results and conclusions for the study at hand with other (independent) reports having the same focus. The decision to transfer results (or not) is based on: (a) the consumer's local perspective, and (b) the external consistency of the results and conclusions.

Combining Qualitative and Quantitative Methods

Trochim (2004) professed that good research requires both qualitative and the quantitative methods. In fact, most qualitative research contains quantification in one form or another. An example is Bloom's (1970) qualitative study of early language development. Though the vast majority of the data was qualitative in nature, Bloom reported frequencies of occurrence (a quantitative measure) for the children's single-word utterances. Trochim (2004) observed that researchers are increasingly interested in blending the qualitative and quantitative traditions to get the advantages of each. *The Office of Behavioral and Social Sciences Research: National Institutes of Health* (OBSSR, 2004) recommended four models for combining qualitative and quantitative approaches within a single study. The four models are as follows:

Technology Note

The internet has emerged as the world's largest electronic archive of written material and a major source for interpersonal exchange, Websites and internet communities such as *chat rooms, listservs,* and *newsgroups* are rich sources of qualitative data, but internet-based research raises some ethical concerns, according to Eysenbach and Till (2001). For example, qualitative researchers may employ online interviews, online focus groups, or online surveys to collect qualitative data. If the online sites are public places, *informed consent* may be unnecessary, but if an online site is deemed to be private, informed consent is clearly required. However, determining whether there is a reasonable expectation of privacy or not for a particular website is not always simple. The internet also presents a challenge for the *confidentiality* of qualitative data. What criteria would you adopt to determine if an online site is private or public? Compare your criteria to Eysenbach and Till's criteria. What would you do to protect the *confidentiality* of online research?

1. *Sequential.* Qualitative models serve for the first stage of knowledge building to discover key issues and elements for subsequent study using formal structured methods. For example, focus groups and preliminary pilot studies are conducted to refine a standardized instrument of clinical assessment for use in a new population or ethnic group.
2. *Parallel.* Some models effectively conduct qualitative methods such as case studies, focused ethnographic observation, or multiple linked indepth interviews (or a combination of these) in tandem with other methods.
3. *Coordinated sub-studies.* Qualitative studies contribute under the umbrella of a larger program project or long-term study.
4. *Integrated.* Methodologically diverse concepts and data are integrated at each stage within the study design to develop a robust evaluation of each emerging finding and set of data.

Culatta, Kovarsky, Theadore, Franklin, and Timler's (2003) study illustrates the *parallel model* for combining qualitative and quantitative approaches within a single study. They adopted the parallel model to study early literacy instruction. Culatta and colleagues (2003) explained as follows:

> Although quantitative procedures were used to evaluate the effectiveness of the literacy instruction in terms of performance measures, qualitative analyses provided information about children's engagement and participation in instructional activities and documented changes in performance over time. (p. 177)

Based on their quantitative results, Culatta and colleagues (2003) concluded that some treatment conditions were better than others. The qualitative results were summed up as: "A qualitative examination of children's participation revealed their affective involvement and engagement in instructional activities" (p. 172). Thus, the combination of qualitative and quantitative methods yielded distinctly different but complementary information about literacy instruction.

A second example of qualitative and quantitative approaches combined in a single study was reported by Strum and Nelson (1997). They described the roles of qualitative and quantitative analyses as follows:

> The 15 classrooms were chosen to permit a rich description of both qualitative and quantitative aspects of formal classroom discourse. The qualitative analysis involved a series of multiple passes through the transcripts to develop a coding system, a series of themes, and eventually, a set of 10 rules to describe the interactions. The quantitative analysis involved compiling data such as numbers of words spoken and numbers of words per T-unit (or C-unit) by both students and teachers at each of the three grade levels. The frequencies of various communicative functions were also examined across grade levels. (Strum & Nelson, 1997, p. 256)

Given the four models for combining qualitative and quantitative approaches within a single study, which of the four models best fits the description provided by Strum and Nelson (1997)? How did combining qualitative and quantitative approaches yield a richer analysis of Strum and Nelson's data?

CASE STUDIES

Case 5.1   Career in Speech-Language Pathology?

Barbara, a graduate student in speech-language pathology, is developing a thesis proposal. Her timeline for completing the thesis is 12 months from today. Barbara and the thesis advisor, Dr. Penny, plan to answer the question: Why do students choose a career in speech-language pathology? What type of qualitative research design or combination of designs do you recommend for Barbara's thesis?

Case 5.2   Focus on AAC

Dr. Hannity is Jean's research mentor at the local university. Jean is a speech-language pathologist at the regional trauma center. Dr. Hannity has assigned Jean to plan and develop a focus group to evaluate a new product for augmentative/alternative communication use. You volunteered to help Jean with the project because you recently completed a research class. What steps will you and Jean follow to organize and conduct the focus group?

Case 5.3   Email or Not to Email

A fellow student, Roy, asked you to participate in an online interview. Roy is completing a requirement for his senior research class, and he plans to conduct unstructured interviews with 10 students as participants. The research question is: What are students' attitudes and opinions about cheating on exams? Roy plans to conduct the interviews solely by email exchanges. What questions should you ask?

Student Exercises

1. What steps would you take to triangulate data sources in a qualitative study with a focus on nonverbal communication?
2. How would you adopt the *sequential model* to plan a qualitative/quantitative study to develop a test of reading fluency for bilingual Asian-American children?
3. Search the professional journals for a recent report that employs the case study method as the principle research design. Is the case study qualitative, quantitative, or a combination of qualitative and quantitative? What proportion of the study is quantitative and what proportion is qualitative?
4. How would you employ *lamination* as a technique to verify your interpretation of data gathered from direct observations of speech-language evaluations?
5. Search the communication disorders journals and identify a qualitative research report. Evaluate the *transferability* of the results and conclusions. What steps did the researchers take to insure transferability of results and conclusions? How would you improve the transferability of the study's results and conclusions?

6 Single-Case Designs in Communication Disorders Research

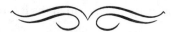

explore (ĭk splôr′) v. to investigate systematically; to make a careful examination or search.

The family of single-case designs includes *simple case studies* and *time-series designs*. The simple case study is typically a thorough description of one or more children or adults and is usually more qualitative than quantitative. Simple case studies lack the controls that are included in experimental designs. Thus, they fall short of the rigorous standards that typify scientific inquiry. However, uncontrolled case studies are an excellent choice when the purpose is to generate ideas. In that sense, uncontrolled case studies may be the genesis of scientific inquiry.

In contrast to simple case studies, *time-series designs* typically include controls that meet the rigorous standards of scientific inquiry. Time-series designs observe a series of behaviors across some period of time, and they permit cause-effect conclusions, though the conclusions are less robust than those from randomized-controlled group designs. For this reason, time-series designs are classified as quasi-experimental designs.

One use of time-series designs is to gather preliminary data before undertaking a randomized-controlled group experiment. In this sense, time-series designs are exploratory in nature. However, time-series designs provide strong evidence for clinical practice—especially when results from several independent studies are combined.

A special instance of time-series designs is known as the *single-case design*—and single-case designs are commonly employed in communication disorders. The unit of analysis in single-case designs is usually a single individual—though it may be a dyad, small group of individuals, or a classroom. When the unit of analysis is a group, the data for analysis may be a group statistic such as a mean, median, or standard deviation, and researchers report individual results along with group results to show that the treatment affected most participants in the same way. The basic sequence of events for a single case design is depicted in the following:

$$O_1 \; O_2 \; O_3 \; I_1 \; O_4 \; O_5 \; O_6$$

The symbol O represents the observation of a dependent variable, and the symbol I represents a one-time intervention. In this case, $O_1 - O_3$ represents observations that take place in a baseline phase—and $O_4 - O_6$ are observations that follow the one-time intervention. More often, interventions are continuously applied throughout the intervention phase. In this case, the basic single-case protocol is illustrated as

$$O_1 \; O_2 \; O_3 \; I_1 \; O_4 \; I_1 \; O_5 \; I_1 \; O_6$$

In this formula, the O_4, O_5, and O_6 observations follow interventions (I_1) throughout the treatment phase. The use of a continuous treatment in single-case designs is typical in communication disorders research. The family of time-series designs includes many variations of the basic designs depicted in the formulas above.

Single-Case Designs Versus Group Designs

Single-case research designs are unlike group research designs in many ways. First, they focus on individual performance, whereas group designs focus on group performance. Second, single-case designs compare different conditions within one participant, whereas group designs compare a treatment group to one or more control groups. For internal validity, group designs rely on the external controls provided by comparison groups or no-treatment control groups, whereas single-case designs rely on comparisons between different conditions or phases.

The comparisons in single-case designs are made by presenting alternative conditions to a participant at different points in time. For example, a treatment may be evaluated by alternating periods of treatment and no-treatment across time. Inferences are made about the treatment in single-case designs based on the patterns of the data across the different conditions. A third way in which single-case and group designs differ regards external validity and the ability to generalize results to the population of interest. Group designs depend on representative samples selected from the population for their external validity, whereas single-case designs depend on replication with additional participants for their external validity. Single-case designs are less rigorous in this regard because replication with two or more participants may suggest that an intervention is applicable to others, but it is not conclusive evidence. Fourth, single-case designs require decision making regarding the course of the study as it progresses, whereas group designs are planned beforehand and carried out with little if any change in the original plan.

The Baseline Phase in Single-Case Designs

Single-case designs begin with systematic observations of an individual's behavior for several sessions before the treatment is introduced. This period of time is known as the *baseline phase* (sometimes referred to as the *pre-treatment phase*). The baseline phase has two purposes: (a) to describe the extent of the individual's problem, or status of the target behavior as it naturally occurs, and (b) to predict future behavior if intervention is not provided. To insure the reliability of measurements and the validity of the baseline, a minimum of 5 to 10 observations are usually prescribed. However, the exact number of observations in the baseline phase depends on the stability or degree of variability of the dependent variable. Observations continue and data are collected until a predictable pattern of behavior is established. If the observed behavior is erratic and no stable pattern emerges, the experiment may conclude with no intervention. If the observed behavior is stable with a predictable trend, an intervention phase is initiated in the next session.

There are four basic types of single-case designs: (a) the A-B-A-B design, (b) the multiple-baseline (changing-baseline) design, (c) the changing-criterion design, and (d) the simultaneous-treatment design. However, many variations or elaborations of these basic designs exist.

The A-B-A Single-Case Design

The A-B-A single-case design is a prototype for single case quasi-experimental research. The A-B-A-B design is an extension of the A-B-A design that adds a B phase to the A-B-A sequence. The A-B-A notation represents a series of three phases that are implemented over time. The first A is an initial baseline phase, wherein the dependent variable is observed in its natural state, and data are collected until a stable baseline is clearly visible or established by statistical analysis procedures. The A phase is important because it is the basis for predicting the natural course of the behavior without intervention of the treatment. The B represents the intervention phase wherein the treatment is first introduced, and the second A represents a second baseline condition wherein the treatment is withdrawn. In its extended form (A-B-A-B), the final B phase is a reintroduction of the intervention. The added B condition in the A-B-A-B design addresses the ethical concern that the experiment may conclude without the benefit of intervention for the participant.

The A-B-A-B design has an additional advantage over the A-B-A design in that it replicates the A-B comparison (A-B + A-B). This internal replication of the A-B sequence provides additional support for a cause-effect relationship between independent (intervention) and dependent (behavioral) variables. Figure 6.1 displays a prototypical A-B-A-B single-case design with four phases and fictitious data from observations of a dependent variable.

The first A phase (A_1) in Figure 6.1 illustrates the measurement of a subject's behavior across 5 sessions. The schedule for baseline probes depends on the nature of the target behavior and other factors, so the 5 sessions may occur in 1 day or over the course of 5 consecutive days at prescribed intervals of time. In this illustration, the data recorded in the A phase are relatively stable with little variation observed from session to session. To conclude that a baseline is stable, the dependent variable should be relatively unchanging across at least three consecutive sessions. This is a critical assumption for time-series designs because it is the basis for predicting the future course of the dependent variable. Once a stable baseline is established, the treatment phase begins with the first session in the B_1 phase and usually continues for 5 or more sessions until the

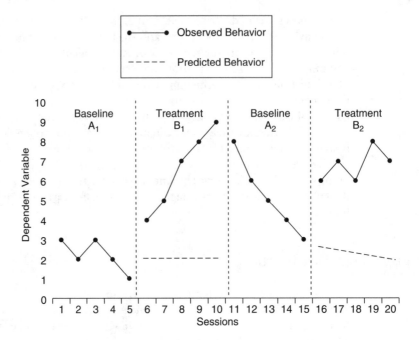

Figure 6.1   A-B-A-B single-case design.

experimenter is satisfied that the effect of the intervention (or non-effect) is evident. The broken line in phase B_1 (Figure 6.1) depicts the prediction inferred by the pattern of observations in phase A_1.

The baseline data in phase A_1 predict that the observed behavior will continue on the same course for future sessions if a treatment is not introduced. This prediction is the basis of comparison, as well as the internal control that provides scientific credibility for the experimental outcome. The solid line in the first treatment phase (B_1) represents the participant's performance across sessions 6–10. The treatment phase may continue for more than 5 sessions depending on the targeted behavior and the observed change (if any) in the participant's performance. The effect of the treatment is inferred by comparing the solid line shown in the treatment phase B_1 to the broken line in the same phase—or, alternatively, the solid line in A_1 to the solid line in B_1. In this case, a visual inspection of the results suggests that the change in behavior during the B_1 phase is not predicted by the baseline data in A_1. This is preliminary evidence for efficacy, but it lacks confirmation.

To test the assumption that the original baseline was an accurate predictor of future performance, a second baseline phase (A_2) is introduced by withdrawing the treatment but continuing to observe the behavior across sessions 11–15. The second A phase (A_2)—sometimes referred to as the *withdrawal phase*—is important because it tests the internal validity of the experiment by ruling out history and maturation effects (nuisance variables) as causes of the change in behavior observed in B_1. If the dependent variable regresses toward the baseline, the experimenters may conclude that the treatment has a causal relationship to the behavior. However, if the dependent variable fails to regress toward the baseline or trends upward in the withdrawal phase A_2, confirmation of a cause-effect relationship is not possible—and the experiment may conclude.

If a regression to baseline effect is observed in A_2, the treatment is reintroduced in the B_2 phase. Again, the course of behavior predicted by the previous phase is illustrated by the broken line in B_2, and the actual behavior observed in phase B_2 is depicted as a solid line. The effect of reintroducing the treatment in phase B_2 is evaluated by comparing the actual performance (solid line) to the predicted performance (broken line). If reintroducing the treatment in phase B_2 results in a change in the dependent variable similar to the change observed in phase B_1, researchers may conclude that the treatment is a cause for the observed change in the behavior. This does not necessarily mean that the intervention is the sole cause of the change because extraneous variables cannot be totally ruled out. However, if extraneous variables are present, their contribution to the change in behavior is probably small.

The A-B-A and A-B-A-B designs include one independent variable (usually a treatment variable) to test the effect of an intervention. However, researchers in communication disorders may want to compare the effects of different treatments on a target behavior. For example, researchers may want to compare the effects of two instructional procedures for teaching reading to young children. A single-case design for testing the effects of two treatment variables is the A-B-A-C single-case design. In this design, the first treatment variable is designated as B, and the second treatment variable is designated as C. The A-B-A-C single-case design is a useful design, but it requires care to avoid *multiple-treatment interference,* which is a serious threat to internal validity.

Multiple-treatment interference is a problem inherent in A-B-A-C single-case designs because the effects of treatment B are likely to carry over to treatment C, thus contaminating the C phase with an unwanted nuisance variable. Multiple-treatment interference is controlled in advance by recruiting additional participants and counterbalancing the order of treatments across subjects. For example, if an A-B-A-C design includes four participants, treatments are counterbalanced across participants as follows: (1) A-B-A-C, (2) A-C-A-B, (3) A-B-A-C, and (4) A-C-A-B. In this case, the experiment's outcome is evaluated as the summative effect of treatments across the four subjects.

Though experimenters may conclude that a treatment was cause for a change in behavior, conclusions based on one individual cannot be generalized to the target population. To provide evidence for the generalization of results to other cases (external validity), direct replication with additional participants is the usual choice. Thus, most single-case experiments in communication disorders include three or more participants.

Replication in Single-Case Designs

In single-case designs (and group designs), *replication* involves repeating the experiment with exactly the same conditions but with different subjects. If the same intervention effect is demonstrated with two or more additional participants, experimenters may conclude that the intervention is effective with a variety of individuals, and this is evidence for external validity. However, the evidence may fall short of proving that the intervention will benefit all children or adults that are like the participants in the study. At best, the successful replication of a single-case experiment suggests that the results can be generalized but is less than conclusive. The best scientific evidence that a particular intervention is applicable to the population of children or adults is achieved by randomized-controlled experiments with (large) representative samples of participants randomly selected from the population. However, the synthesis of results from small n studies, such as single-case experiments is strong evidence as well.

Example of the A-B-A-B Single-Case Design in Communication Disorders

To study the effects on children's speech rates when their mothers talked more slowly, two researchers (Guitar & Marchinkoski, 2001) adopted an A-B-A-B single-case design. Their units of analysis were 6 mother-child dyads—3 boys and 3 girls, 3–4 years of age. The researchers manipulated the speech rates of the mothers (independent variable) in the intervention phases (B_1, B_2) of the A-B-A-B design, and the mothers' natural speech rates were observed in the baseline phases. In the first B phase (intervention), the mothers were trained to use a slow speech rate. The dependent variable was speech rate as measured in syllables per minute. Each phase in their A-B-A-B design was 10 minutes long with 8 probes or measurements of the dependent variable. The researchers concluded that 5 of the 6 children reduced their speech rates when their mothers spoke more slowly. However, their conclusions were tentative because speech rates varied widely in some conditions. In other words, they failed to achieve a stable baseline with some cases. The researchers suggested that a replication of their study would benefit from extending the length of phases to achieve stable speech rates.

Visual Inspection Versus Statistical Tests

To conclude that a treatment is effective in a single-case design, researchers may choose visual inspection, statistical procedures, or a combination of both visual inspection and statistics (usually the best choice). Visual inspection is the initial choice of most researchers because the phases in single-case designs are easily graphed, and changes (or no changes) in the dependent variable are readily apparent. However, *visual analyses* are subjective and interrater agreement regarding the presence or absence of a treatment effect in visual analyses typically averages 60 percent or less according to Robey, Schultz, Crawford, and Sinner (1999). Thus, the use of visual inspection alone to judge treatment effects in single-case designs is not a reliable method of analysis.

Technology Note

Statistical tools are useful for analyzing trends in time-series designs. Statistical software packages such as MINITAB and SPSS include trend analysis and autocorrelation functions for analyzing data in time-series designs. An online resource is Dr. Paul Jones' Single-Case Research and Statistical Analysis web pages. The Jones website includes statistical analysis tools with autocorrelation, chi square, nonparametric, time series, and t-test options. Program instructions on the website include features, general functions, and data entry procedures. A "personal version" of the statistical analysis program is available for offline data processing. The Single-Case Research and Statistical Analysis website is located at: *http://www.unlv.edu/faculty/pjones/singlecase/scsainst.htm.*

Because of the shortcomings inherent in visual analyses, researchers utilize statistical tests such as analysis of variance (ANOVA), t tests, and the standardized effect size (ES). The problem with using ANOVA and t-test procedures with time-series data is that they assume the data for analysis are independent (unrelated to one another). However, because the data in time-series designs are collected from one participant, they are not independent. Statisticians refer to this form of dependence across observations as *temporal autocorrelation.*

For this reason, ANOVA and t-test procedures may be subject to error when applied to time-series designs. The result is questionable validity. Alternative procedures such as *Interrupted Time Series Analyses* (ITSA), and its variant ITSACORR, yield a test of overall change, a test of change in slope, and a test of change in level (Robey et al., 1999). The ITSA and ITSACORR procedures account for the correlated nature of the data and yield a meaningful statistic (F) that tests the null hypothesis of overall change.

The *effect size (ES) statistic* is not a test of the null hypothesis, but it yields a measure of the overall magnitude of a change. An estimation of effect size for time-series data is relatively easy to compute. The standardized effect size (ES) is derived by the formula shown below (cf. Faith, Allison, & Gorman, 1997).

$$ES = \frac{\overline{X}_B - \overline{X}_A}{S_A}$$

$$\text{where} \quad S_A = \frac{1}{n-1} \sum (x_i - \bar{x})^2$$

The subscripts A and B designate baseline and intervention phases respectively. The mean $(\overline{X})$ is the average for baseline (A) and intervention (B) data, and S is the standard deviation that is calculated from data in the baseline phase. If there is no variability observed in the baseline phase, the effect size cannot be estimated. The effect sizes derived from single-case designs are not the same as the effect sizes computed in group research designs, so they are not comparable.

The Multiple-Baseline
Single-Case Design

The *multiple-baseline single-case design* (also known as a *changing-baseline design*) is pictured as a series of A-B designs stacked on top of one another with each baseline phase progressively longer. There can be three or more baselines, and each baseline represents a *target variable*. The multiple-baseline design includes a treatment variable and three or more target variables. Target variables are chosen carefully because they must be independent of one another. In other words, a change in the treated variable should not be accompanied by a change in an untreated variable.

The multiple-baseline design is a flexible design in that it can simultaneously analyze three or more target behaviors. It also avoids the ethical concern regarding withdrawal of treatment because no withdrawal of treatment is needed. The multiple-baseline design is also an alternative when an A-B-A design is not possible because a dependent variable does not respond to withdrawal of the treatment because of carry-over or long-lasting effects of the treatment on the dependent variable—the generalized effects problem.

Though multiple-baseline designs have some advantages, they also have disadvantages relative to A-B-A designs. First, the multiple-baseline design is weaker than the A-B-A design because the controlling effects of the treatment variable on the dependent variable are not directly demonstrated as they are in the intervention and withdrawal phases of the A-B-A design. Second, multiple-baseline designs require a multitude of data collection over an extended period of time. Thus, the multiple-baseline design requires substantial resources for planning, implementing, and insuring the cooperation of participants.

The multiple-baseline design includes three or more *target variables* with their respective baselines. The target variables may be any one of three types: (a) different *behaviors* for one participant observed in one setting or, alternatively, the sum of responses for more than one participant such as a dyad, small group of individuals, or classroom observed in one setting, (b) different *participants* who are observed in one setting exhibiting one behavior, or (c) different *settings* with one participant and one behavior. Following collection of the baseline data, the treatment variable is introduced to each of the target variables in turn (behaviors, participants, or settings). The introduction of the treatment variable to the second and third target variables is triggered by a predetermined level of performance. For example, if the dependent variable increases by a predetermined level of 50 percent, the treatment is applied to the second target variable while, the first target variable continues to be treated and so on. Figure 6.2 illustrates a prototypical multiple-baseline design with two phases (A-B), multiple tiers, and fictitious data from observations of a dependent variable.

The symbol *A* represents the baseline phase, wherein the dependent variable is observed in its natural state, and data are collected until a stable baseline is established. In this case, baseline data are collected concurrently on the three baselines. The symbol *B* represents the intervention phase, wherein the treatment is introduced. Each of the tiers represents one target variable. The treatment is applied to each target variable but at different points in time. Thus, the treatment is applied to the first target variable and when the response reaches a predetermined level, the treatment is applied to the second target variable and then the third target behavior, until the treatment has been applied to all of the target behaviors. The multiple-baseline single-case design demonstrates a treat-

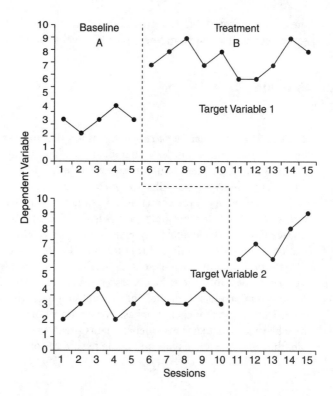

Figure 6.2   Multiple-baseline single-case design.

ment effect by showing that the response changes whenever the treatment is introduced at the different points in time.

Example of the Multiple-Baseline Single-Case Design in Communication Disorders

To study the effect of typicality of exemplars on naming ability, two researchers (Kiran & Thompson, 2003) adopted a multiple-baseline across behaviors single-case design. The *behaviors* in this case were different levels of typicality (typical, intermediate, and atypical) for specific semantic categories. For example, "parrot" was a typical referent in the bird category, but "penguin" was an atypical referent. The units of analysis were four adult participants with fluent aphasia—3 females and 1 male, 63–75 years of age. The researchers employed a semantic feature treatment as their intervention. The dependent variable was the number of items named correctly. The number of probes during the intervention phases ranged from 6 to 11. The researchers reported that 3 of the 4 participants demonstrated a stable baseline which the researchers operationally defined as less than 2 points fluctuation across sessions. The researchers observed positive changes in the dependent variable (naming ability) after treatment was introduced and also observed generalization from one typicality level to another.

The Changing-Criterion
Single-Case Design

The *changing-criterion single-case design* is another time-series design that employs baseline and intervention phases to demonstrate a treatment effect while controlling extraneous influences. The changing-criterion design is especially well suited for solving clinical problems where skills are practiced and achieved gradually, not abruptly. The sequence of events in the changing-criterion design is A-B_1-B_2-B_3 where A is the baseline phase, and the intervention phase B is divided into several subphases. An optional phase—known as a *maintenance phase*—may follow the intervention phase. A prototypical changing-criterion design that includes fictitious data is pictured in Figure 6.3.

As is typical with single-case designs, the baseline phase of the changing-criterion design continues until the subject's responses are stabilized across three or more sessions. An intervention phase is divided into several subphases that include gradually changing criteria. The criterion for each subphase is the number of responses that need to be performed to achieve a particular consequence that is predetermined by the investigator. For example, the consequence may be a tangible reward of some sort that is awarded on a regular

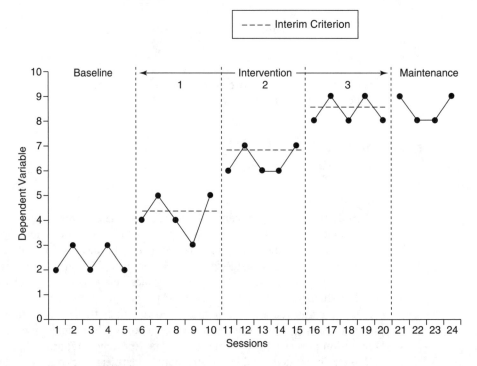

Figure 6.3   Changing-criterion single-case design.

schedule within each session. In the changing-criterion design, the criterion is gradually changed at the end of each subphase of the intervention. The criterion is typically increased so that the subject must demonstrate a slightly greater performance to earn the reward. The criterion is changed throughout the intervention phase until a terminal goal is achieved.

In the changing-criterion design, the treatment effect is demonstrated if the subject's performances match the criteria as they are changed. If performances closely match the criteria, the investigator may conclude that the intervention is responsible for changes in the dependent variable—and extraneous variables are not. If the intervention is shown to be effective, the investigator may continue to observe the subject's behavior in an additional phase—known as a *maintenance phase*—across several sessions or more. The purpose of the maintenance phase is to determine the degree of carry-over for the treatment effect.

A disadvantage of the changing-criterion single-case design is the possibility of ambiguity if the subject's performance does not closely follow the positive changes in the criterion. A variation of the changing-criterion design includes *mini-reversal phases,* wherein the investigator makes bidirectional changes in the interim criteria. In this case, the treatment effect is demonstrated if the responses match the criteria as they change direction. Overall, the changing-criterion design is appropriate for establishing a functional relationship between a treatment and behavior, but it requires intensive planning and careful implementation for success.

The Simultaneous-Treatment Single-Case Design

The purpose of the simultaneous-treatment single-case design is to compare the effects of alternate treatments on a dependent variable. It exposes one participant to two different treatments at the same time. To control for extraneous influences, such as history and maturation effects, the order of treatments is counterbalanced. For example, the two treatments are alternated 1–2 on one day, 2–1 on the next day, and so on. In this case, the participant is exposed to both treatments in the same day but in different sessions. A prototypical simultaneous-treatment single-case design with fictitious data is displayed in Figure 6.4.

The baseline data are collected in both sessions prior to introducing the treatment. Once stable baselines are established, the intervention phase B begins with the first treatment introduced in session one and the second treatment introduced in session two. The presentation of treatments is subsequently counterbalanced from day to day for the remainder of intervention. If one treatment is shown to be superior to the other treatment, the superior treatment may be continued in both sessions during phase C. The intervention is concluded when the treatment effect is clearly demonstrated, and an optional phase D begins. Phase D is a maintenance phase, wherein the investigators observe the treatment's carryover effect.

The simultaneous-treatment design is an alternative design for comparing the effects of two treatments applied concurrently, but it has some limitations. First, the design may include additional treatments, but it is difficult to balance more than two treatments at a time. Therefore, two simultaneous treatments are optimal. Second, *multiple-treatment interference* is a threat to internal validity. The design depends on treatments that have little or no carryover effect from treatment to treatment, and multiple-treatment interference may be difficult to detect.

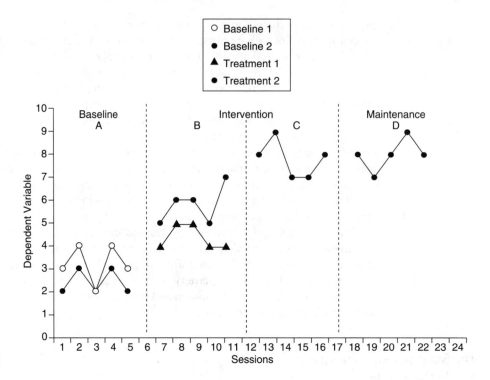

Figure 6.4   Simultaneous-treatment single-case design.

Overall, the simultaneous-treatment single-case design is an alternative time-series design especially suited to comparing two or more treatments. However, it requires careful planning and implementation to ensure valid results.

Example of the Simultaneous-Treatment Single-Case Design in Communication Disorders

Meline, Gonzalez, Florez-Sabo, and Hinojosa (2004) employed a variation of the simultaneous-treatment single-case design. The Meline et al. research team examined the effects of two different treatments (modeling and paired reading) on third-grade children's reading performances—both reading accuracy and reading rate. Meline et al. (2004) counterbalanced reading passages as well as the two treatments of the independent variable.

Figure 6.5 displays Meline et al.'s (2004) results for one of the four participants. In this example, the dependent variable was reading rate. Baseline data are recorded in the A phase, and treatment data are recorded in the B phase. The baseline data (sessions 1–4) were horizontally stable, indicating a stable baseline. However, the overall slope across

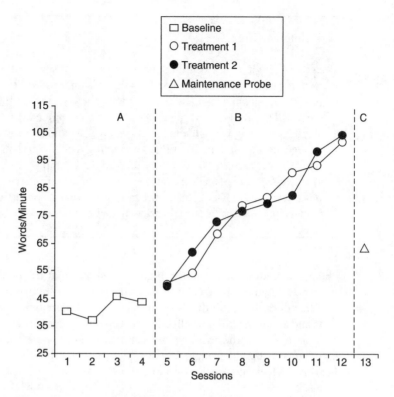

Figure 6.5 Simultaneous-treatment single-case design.

sessions 1–12 departed significantly from the horizontal plane, thus suggesting a treatment effect. The difference between the modeling and paired reading treatments was not significant.

Another indicator of treatment effects is known as the "percentage of non-overlapping data" (PND). The PND is calculated as the percentage of data values in the treatment phase (phase B) that exceeds the largest data value in the baseline phase (phase A). In Meline et al.'s (2004) case, 100 percent of the data in phase B exceeded the largest value in phase A. Thus, the treatment was evaluated as "very effective." Typically, a PND > 90 percent is interpreted as "very effective"; a PND between 70 and 90 percent is "moderately effective"; and a PND < 70 percent suggests a weak effect or no effect at all. The PND is usually a reliable indicator of treatment effectiveness, but it is not a reliable indicator in every case (cf. Scruggs & Mastropieri, 2001). For example, the PND metric is not sensitive to slope changes, and it is influenced by the number of observations.

In addition to the usual baseline and treatment phases, Meline et al. (2004) introduced a maintenance probe (phase C): (a) to test carry-over effects with a novel reading passage, and (b) to test the possible effect of "repeated readings." Though Meline et al. (2004) counterbalanced their presentation of reading passages in the treatment phase, *repeated readings* (a potential nuisance variable) may have contributed to the observed

---

Technology Note

Because single-case research depends on visual displays of data for its interpretation, the production of suitable line graphs is important. There are numerous computer software packages with tools for creating graphs; however, most are not suitable for single-case designs. An excellent resource for creating line graphs for single-case designs is a technical article by Carr and Burkholder (1998). They described step-by-step instructions for creating *A-B-A-B* and *multiple-baseline* graphs with *Microsoft Excel*. The Carr and Burkholder examples were based on *Excel 97 for Windows/NT* and *MacOS* operating systems, but their instructions are adaptable to newer versions of *Excel*. An advantage of preparing graphs in a spreadsheet program is that the data can be stored and analyzed in the same program.

---

change in reading performance. Figure 6.5 shows that the participant's reading performance declined in phase C but remained significantly above the baseline performance.

What does the result displayed in phase C of Figure 6.5 suggest about carry-over effects and about the possible effects of repeated readings? How could Meline et al. (2004) have strengthened the outcome for their maintenance phase? How would you employ the simultaneous-baseline single case design to compare the effects of two different assistive hearing devices on speech discrimination?

Conclusion: Single-Case Designs in Communication Disorders

Single-case quasi-experimental designs are underutilized in communication disorders research. It may be that veteran researchers and prospective researchers are less familiar with the elements of single-case designs than with traditional group designs. Another factor may be that some researchers view single-case designs as inadequate for answering research questions. When single-case controlled designs are properly planned and implemented, they are legitimate alternatives to other experimental designs in communication disorders and are superior in some respects. A particular strength of single-case controlled designs is the focus on individuals, whereas a limitation is the inability to extend results to the target population. An additional strength of single-case designs is the ability to examine treatment effects in a maintenance phase, where carry-over effects can be evaluated. The maintenance of treatment effects is a somewhat neglected area of study in communication disorders.

Single-case designs are flexible in their applications and are available in a variety of basic types, including A-B-A-(B), multiple-baseline, changing-criterion, and simultaneous-treatment designs. For in-depth study of single-case designs and their many applications, Hersen and Barlow (1976), Kratochwill (1978), and Franklin, Allison, and Gorman (1997) are representative of the many textbooks devoted to the topic.

CASE STUDIES

Case 6.1   Problem of Limited Resources

Ms. McCarthy, a clinician-researcher, and Professor Schmitt are planning a research study to investigate the effect of a novel treatment on 6-year-old children's phonological behaviors. They have limited resources in terms of numbers of potential participants and time. As a consultant, what research design do you recommend to Ms. McCarthy and Professor Schmitt, and what are the benefits and limitations of following your recommendations?

Case 6.2   Quest for Evidence of Maintenance

A team of four researchers is planning a collaboration to investigate the short-term and long-term carry-over effects of a proven intervention for reading comprehension skills. What are your recommendations for a plan to achieve their research goals, and what benefits and limitations are related to your recommendations?

Case 6.3   Balancing Ethics with Scientific Inquiry

Mr. Scott, a clinician-researcher, and Dr. Salinas, a veteran research scientist, are collaborators in a study that aims to explore the effects of training on certain conversational behaviors. They planned to implement an A-B-A single case design, but objections were raised by the *Institutional Review Board,* as well as from teachers of the prospective participants. What are the researchers' alternative choices in this case?

Student Exercises

1. Search the communication disorders journals for a research report that includes a single-case quasi-experimental design and evaluate the investigators' implementation of the design including baseline and intervention phases.
2. Locate an example of an A-B-A or A-B-A-B single case design in the communication disorders research literature. How did the researchers address the issue of external validity? How could they have evaluated carry-over of the treatment effect?
3. Evaluate the investigators' conclusions in a research report that employs a single-case design—such as an A-B-A-B or multiple-baseline design. How are the researchers' conclusions related to the results? Are the research conclusions accurately stated?
4. Search the communication disorders journals for a research report that includes a comparison of two groups of participants in a group design. Explain how the investigators might have used a single-case design to answer their research questions, and discuss the advantages and disadvantages of each design choice (group vs. single-case).
5. Locate a single-case design in a research report and evaluate the researchers' interpretation of changes in the dependent variable from baseline to intervention, or intervention to baseline. Calculate an effect size (ES) for one of their baselines and interpret the result. HINT: You can estimate the values of the dependent variable from the visual displays of results. This task is easier if the figures are enlarged on a copier.

7 Alternative Designs in Communication Disorders Research

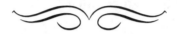

observe   (əb-zûrv′) v. to contemplate, detect, discern, discover, distinguish, examine, inspect, perceive, recognize, study, survey, view.

In experimental research designs, the subjects' behaviors are observed in response to a planned treatment. If a change in behavior is observed, the treatment is presumed to be the *cause*, and the change in behavior is presumed to be the *effect*. The goal of experimental research is to evaluate the effect of a treatment, and experimental research designs permit conclusions about causality. However, not all research endeavors aim to evaluate cause and effect. Many research endeavors seek to describe subjects' behaviors with no attempt to change the behaviors. When causality is not central to the research purpose, researchers choose from a variety of alternative designs. Common designs in communication disorders include: (a) case studies, (b) ethnographic research, (c) historical research, (d) correlational research, (e) developmental research, and (f) survey research designs.

Why do researchers need so many different designs? Why not answer all the questions in communication disorders with one or two research designs? The many research designs in communication disorders are uniquely suited for answering specific questions. Each research design has distinctive features.

Distinctive Features of Alternative Designs

Case Study and Ethnographic Designs

Case study and ethnographic research types are distinguished by their thorough descriptions of one or more participant's traits and behaviors. The *case study* approach targets a single participant, whereas *ethnographic research* usually targets a group of individuals who share a common bond, such as a specific disability or cultural traits. The case study approach is especially suited for describing unusual clinical cases that manifest rare diseases or conditions. A case in point is Cox, Lee, Carey, and Minor's (2003) description of a patient who presented auditory and vestibular symptoms associated with a rare syndrome. The prominent features of the syndrome were vertigo and an opening in the bone above the semicircular canals. In an application of the ethnographic approach, O'Neil-Pirozzi (2003) studied education, health problems, and speech-language abilities of 25 homeless mothers and their children.

The results of case studies and ethnographic research may have immediate clinical applications. They also provide direction for future studies. What is a possible clinical application from the Cox et al. (2003) case study? What ideas for future research may come from O'Neil-Pirozzi's (2003) ethnographic study?

Historical Research

Historical research is unique in that it collects data for analysis from existing records. The purpose of historical research is to construct theories and develop hypotheses based on the historical evidence. For example, researchers collect data from clinical records to evaluate clinical outcomes. Who are the participants in historical research? Is informed consent necessary? What are the strengths and weaknesses of historical research? How does historical research contribute to future studies?

Correlational Research

Correlational research designs aim to describe the relationship between two or more variables. When two variables are tested and determined to have a relationship, they are said to be *correlated*. The term *correlation* is derived from "co-relate," and it refers to the relationship between two or more variables. *AllPsych ONLINE* (2004) reported that the correlation is one of the easiest descriptive procedures to understand and one of the most widely used in research.

The correlational research question is written as follows: Is there a (statistically significant) relationship between variable A and variable B? Correlations have *direction* (positive or negative) and *strength* (weak or strong). The strength and direction of a correlation are depicted in the following.

Perfect (-) Correlation		Perfect (+) Correlation
	No Correlation	
-1	0	+1
Negative Correlation		Positive Correlation

In the case of positive correlations, individuals score high (or low) on one variable and score similarly on the other variable. In the case of negative correlations, individuals score high (or low) on one variable and score inversely on the other variable. Correlations also differ in their strength. The strength of a relationship can be anywhere between 0 and ± 1.00.

Typically, correlations do not imply causality because they do not meet the requirements—especially the requirement that no other variable can account for the cause. To illustrate the complexity of correlations and causality, consider an example from *AllPsych* ONLINE (2004). Correlations were reported as follows:

1. There is a positive correlation between ice cream consumption and drowning.
2. There is a positive correlation between ice cream consumption and murder.
3. There is a positive correlation between ice cream consumption and boating accidents.
4. There is a positive correlation between ice cream consumption and shark attacks.

Does ice cream cause people to drown? Does ice cream cause murder? Does ice cream cause boating accidents? Does ice cream cause shark attacks? In reality, ice cream is positively correlated with the other variables because of a third variable. What is the unaccounted variable? The third variable is *weather*—because as the weather becomes warmer, more ice cream is consumed. How does weather account for increases in drowning, murder, boating accidents, and shark attacks?

Thus, correlational procedures are typically not employed to imply causality. However, if a strong relationship is found between variables, special correlational designs can evaluate causality. The most common procedure is known as *path analysis*. Path analysis is based on the regression model. *Regression* refers to the degree to which one variable can be predicted from another variable. The regression model includes criterion variables and predictor variables. The *criterion variable* is what is being predicted, and the *predictor variable* is what is used to make the prediction. On the basis of regression results, researchers determine which of a number of pathways connects one variable with another.

Other types of correlational designs include multiple regression and factor analysis. The *multiple regression* procedure extends regression and prediction by adding several more variables. *Factor analysis* is a statistical procedure that involves a large number of correlated variables and seeks to identify a common underlying factor.

Developmental Research

A design for studying development over a long period of time is known as *developmental research*. The goal of developmental research is to identify developmental trends by observing a particular behavior over months or years. Developmental research designs do not specify causality.

Survey Research

Survey research aims to describe the attitudes, beliefs, or behaviors of a particular population of individuals. Surveys are used by pollsters and marketers to gather opinions and to evaluate consumer behaviors. An example in communication disorders is the mail survey reported by Blood, Ridenour, Thomas, Qualls, and Hammer (2002). The research team employed a survey to evaluate job satisfaction of speech-language pathologists (SLPs) in public schools. They concluded that a majority of SLPs were satisfied with their jobs based on a 60 percent return rate (number of mail surveys returned). In similar fashion, Emanuel (2002) mailed a questionnaire about auditory processing diagnostic practices to all licensed audiologists in Maryland. Emanuel (2002) reported a 55 percent response rate.

Correlational Research in Communication Disorders

Researchers in communication disorders choose *correlational research designs* to explore relationships between two variables or many variables. According to Kerlinger (1973), "[the purpose of correlational research] is to discover significant variables in the field situation, to discover relations among variables, and to lay groundwork for later, more systematic and rigorous testing of hypotheses."

In communication disorders, a correlation of 0.30 is usually meaningful, and a correlation of 0.70 is nearly always meaningful. A correlation means that the measurement of one variable explains something about the measurement of the other variable.

The statistical analysis in correlational designs depends on what are known as *correlation coefficients*. The *Pearson product-moment correlation* yields a correlation coefficient (r) based on continuously measured data. The assumptions that are necessary to use the Pearson product-moment correlation are as follows:

1. The measures are approximately normally distributed.
2. The variances of the two measures are similar.
3. The relationship is linear.
4. The sample is representative of the population.
5. The variables are measured on an interval or ratio scale.

Some measurements in communication disorders are ordinal scale (such as ratings). In these cases, the appropriate correlational procedure is the *Spearman rank correlation*. The formulas for the Pearson product-moment and Spearman rank correlations are included in most basic statistics books. The correlational procedures are also included in most statistical software applications, such as *SPSS, SYSTAT,* and *Minitab*.

Technology Note

A cousin to Charles Darwin, Francis Galton (1812–1911) established a laboratory to collect human statistics circa 1885. Galton was the first to use correlational procedures to measure the relationships between human features. He chose the symbol r as his index for correlation. In the course of studying human features, Galton collected impressions of fingers in his lab. He determined that the patterns of loops, whorls, and arches could be used to identify individuals. His discovery was adopted by Scotland Yard in 1901.

A statistic that is closely related to the correlation coefficient is known as the *index of determination* (r^2). The index of determination is simply the arithmetic square of the correlation coefficient. It is interpreted as the proportion of variance in B that is attributable to A. In other words, the index of determination expresses the degree of variance that is shared by two variables. The more two variables have in common—the better the prediction of one variable from the measurement of the other variable. A graph of two variables with shared variance is illustrated in Figure 7.1.

The variables A and B in Figure 7.1 have a relatively small amount of variance in common. Shared variance is indicated by the degree of overlap between circles. If perfectly correlated, two variables would have 100 percent of their variances in common, and the circles would be perfectly superimposed.

In a collaborative effort, Condouris, Meyer, and Tager-Flisberg (2003) investigated the relationship between scores on standardized tests such as the *Clinical Evaluation of Language Fundamentals* (CELF) and measures of spoken language such as mean length of utterance (MLU). They chose a correlational research design to study relationships between 11 different variables. Their research participants included 7 girls and 37 boys with autism. Condouris et al. (2003) reported a total of 55 correlation coefficients. The correlation coefficients ranged from a low of 0.21 (no statistical significance) to a high of 0.92 (statistically significant). Statistical significance of correlation coefficients is evaluated by the t-test. The indexes of determination (r^2) for these correlation coefficients are as follows:

$$0.21 = (0.21)^2 = 0.04$$
$$0.92 = (0.92)^2 = 0.85$$

In one case, 85 percent of the variance was shared by two of the variables studied, and 4 percent of the variance was shared in the other case. Condouris et al. (2003) concluded their study with clinical recommendations based on the correlational results. What does 85 percent shared variance tell you about the two variables? What does 4 percent shared variance tell you about the other two variables?

A second case example is a correlational study reported by Walden and Walden (2004). According to Walden and Walden (2004), "This study attempted to identify audiometric or other patient-related variables that can be obtained prior to hearing aid dispensing, which may be used to predict success with amplification in everyday living" (p. 344). The researchers specified criterion and predictor variables, gathered measurements, and calculated correlation coefficients. Walden and Walden (2004) concluded their study as follows:

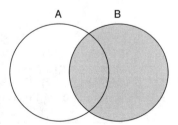

Figure 7.1   Shared variance.

> **Technology Note**
>
> Correlational research designs require statistical analysis tools to compute the correlation coefficients and to test statistical significance. Statistical analysis tools for correlation are readily available in commercial software packages such as MINITAB, SPSS, and Microsoft Excel. Statistical analysis tools including Pearson's Correlation Coefficient are also available as freeware or shareware. Commercial software such as Microsoft Excel typically includes a worksheet with individual cells where the data are entered. Excel includes an Analysis ToolPak that is accessed by clicking Data Analysis on the Tools menu. If Data Analysis is not available on Excel's Tools menu, the Analysis ToolPak add-in program must be installed. Commercial software packages typically include help screens with examples for guidance.

The unaided and aided signal-to-noise ratio (SNR) loss on the QuickSIN test provided the best predictors of hearing aid success in daily living. However, much of this predictive relationship appeared attributable to the patient's age. (p. 342)

Inasmuch as chronological age proved to be an unwanted variable, the researchers utilized a procedure that statistically removed age from the correlation between predictor and criterion variables.

A variable that is measured during the course of a study can be statistically removed after the fact. The statistical procedure that accomplishes this feat is known as the *partial correlation,* so named because it partials (removes) the effect of an unwanted variable. Once age was removed, Walden and Walden (2004) reported that the correlation coefficients diminished and were no longer statistically significant. The researchers concluded as follows: "It appears, therefore, that much of the predictive relationship between the QuickSIN and hearing aid success in everyday life is attributable to the effects of age" (p. 349).

Nathan, Stackhouse, Goulandris, and Snowling (2004) investigated the relationship between speech difficulties and early literacy skills. Their subjects were 47 children from 4 to 7 years of age. The research team employed *path analysis* to investigate developmental relationships between spoken and written language abilities in 4- to 7-year-old children. Based on their results, Nathan et al. (2004) concluded that age-4 language skills were important precursors of reading and spelling abilities at age 6.

Developmental Research in Communication Disorders

Developmental research designs repeatedly measure behaviors over a period of time in order to record developmental trends. The independent variable in developmental studies is *maturation*—whereas the dependent variable is whatever behavior or trait the researchers choose to study. Maturation may be operationally defined as chronological age, but the underlying attributes are the physical and mental changes that take place over time. The basic developmental research types include: (a) longitudinal research, (b) cross-sectional research, and (c) semi-longitudinal research. Each of the three developmental research types purport to accomplish the same task, but each has properties that distinguish it from the others.

The Longitudinal Research Design

Longitudinal research designs observe the same participants over an extended period of time. Longitudinal studies are typically 1 year or more in length. The exact length of a longitudinal study depends on: (a) the nature of the behaviors or traits to be studied, and (b) the goals established by the researchers. To conduct a longitudinal study, researchers develop a plan that specifies the length of the study and the intervals for measurements. For example, a longitudinal study might be 2 years in length with measurements of the dependent variable at 2-week intervals. A research plan of this sort requires a total of 52 observations over the 2-year period. Longitudinal research designs follow the same participants from the beginning of the study to its conclusion. This is a strength that is unique to longitudinal research, but it is also a limitation.

Limitations in Longitudinal Research. Two limitations are inherent in longitudinal research designs. First, the length of longitudinal studies increases the risk of losing participants, and *subject attrition* is a known threat to internal validity. Longitudinal research designs are especially vulnerable in this regard. Because of the length of longitudinal studies, there is a significant risk that one or more participants will leave the geographic area or choose to withdraw from the study for personal reasons. Second, longitudinal studies require substantial human resources and finances to sustain the study for its duration.

Case Example: Longitudinal Research in Communication Disorders. An example of longitudinal research in communication disorders is the collaborative effort by Catts, Fey, Tomblin, and Zhang (2002). They examined reading outcomes for 570 children with language impairments. Catts and colleagues (2002) began their research effort with a sample of 604 participants, but 34 of the 604 participants were lost to attrition. Data were collected in kindergarten, second, and fourth grades. Thus, their study spanned a period of nearly five years. In general, Catts et al. (2002) concluded that children identified as language-impaired in kindergarten were at high risk for reading problems in the second and fourth grades. Was their attrition rate for subjects high or low? An alternative design that addresses the limitations inherent in longitudinal studies but retains the features of developmental research is known as *cross-sectional research*.

The Cross-Sectional Research Design

Cross-sectional designs significantly lessen the threat of subject attrition and reduce the demand on resources. Rather than observe the same participants over an extended period of time, cross-sectional designs include several different groups of participants with each group representing a different point along the developmental continuum. The time period for observation is typically as short as one day—or several weeks.

Limitations in Cross-Sectional Research.   The cross-sectional approach to developmental research saves time and other resources but suffers a limitation of another kind. Longitudinal designs risk a loss of participants, but cross-sectional designs are relatively safe in that regard because of the shorter time period. However, cross-sectional designs include a threat to internal validity known as *nonequivalence*. Because cross-sectional designs include groups with different chronological ages, subjects must be carefully matched to insure equivalence in all respects except age. Cross-sectional designs are inherently weak because observations are snapshots rather than ongoing analyses of behavior. Given this limitation and the threat of nonequivalence, most researchers in communication disorders employ the semi-longitudinal approach to developmental studies.

The Semi-Longitudinal Research Design

Semi-longitudinal research designs combine features of both longitudinal and cross-sectional approaches. The semi-longitudinal approach requires more time to complete than cross-sectional designs but less than longitudinal designs. It includes two or more groups of participants who represent different points on the developmental continuum similar to the selection of participants in cross-sectional designs. The semi-longitudinal approach differs from the cross-sectional approach in that it follows participants for an extended period of time such as 3–12 months. The semi-longitudinal approach is the most popular design for studying developmental changes in communication disorders because it combines the best features of cross-sectional and longitudinal designs.

Limitations in Semi-Longitudinal Research.   *Group equivalency* is a threat to the internal validity of semi-longitudinal studies—but the threat is lessened by the longitudinal component of the design. The semi-longitudinal approach is not as economical as the cross-sectional design but is more economical than the longitudinal approach. Overall, the semi-longitudinal design is a compromise approach that combines features of cross-sectional and longitudinal designs.

Case Examples: Semi-Longitudinal Research in Communication Disorders.   Williams and Elbert (2003) chose a semi-longitudinal design to study phonological development in five late-talking children. They followed two participants at 22 months of age for a period of 10 months and three participants at 30–31 months of age for a period of 12 months. Williams and Elbert collected monthly language samples from each of the five participants. They reported that three of the five participants resolved late onset of speech by 35 months of age, but two participants did not. What was the total duration of the Williams and Elbert (2003) study? What was the advantage of their design over a cross-sectional design?

A second case example is Preisser, Hodson, and Paden's (1988) study of children's normal phonological development from 18 months to 29 months of age. The researchers recruited a total of 60 children with 20 children in each of three groups: 18-month, 22-month, and 26-month age groups. Participants were observed at preplanned intervals over a period of 3 months, so that phonological development was observed in group one from 18–21 months, group two from 22–25 months, and group three from 26–29 months.

As a result, Preisser et al. (1988) recorded changes in phonological development over a span of 11 months; however, the task was completed in 3 months. To accomplish the same task, a longitudinal study would span 11 months. How did Preisser et al. (1988) establish equivalence between the three groups of children? Why not employ a longitudinal design in this case?

The Survey Research Design

The goal of survey research is to investigate the characteristics of a population by collecting representative samples. If each and every member of a population is surveyed, the result is known as a *census*. To obtain a *census*, researchers must identify every member of a population and collect observations from each member. A census is rarely undertaken because costs are prohibitive. For these reasons, researchers rely on samples to generalize results to populations, but the quality of a sample affects the quality of the *inference*.

Sampling Issues in Survey Research Designs

There are many types of sampling methods. The basic method is known as *simple random sampling*. To achieve an unbiased sample, researchers must insure that every member of a population has an equal chance of being included in the sample. The simple random sampling method includes two steps: (a) identify the members of the population—such as all speech-language pathologists working in schools, and (b) randomly select a sample of members from the population. *Fairness* is an important consideration in sampling research, and *bias* is a threat to the fairness of a sample. There are three common sources of bias in samples: (a) failure to identify all members of the population, (b) choosing a sample based on convenience—such as students in a class or patients in a clinic, and (c) constituting a sample from volunteers. In the latter case, the sample may be biased if participants volunteer for personal reasons such as financial need or other reasons that make them fundamentally different from nonvolunteers.

No matter how much care is taken to achieve a representative sample from the population, some sampling error results from simple random sampling. However, sampling error can be minimized by gathering a sample of adequate size. Thus, in a population with 1,000 members, a random sample of 100 participants is probably adequate to generalize results to the population. However, a random sample of 10 participants from the same population contains too much sampling error to allow inferences to the population. Sampling error is reduced by employing what is known as the *stratified sampling method*. The stratified sampling procedure is combined with simple random sampling to achieve a quality sample. The stratified sampling method divides the population into logical divisions to insure that each of the divisions—also known as *strata*—is fairly represented in the sample. For example, the United States is sometimes divided into several geographic regions (strata) to insure that each region is fairly represented in a sample. To insure that a sample matches the proportion of males and females in the population, males and females are identified and sampled in proportions that match the population proportions (e.g., 105 males per 100 females < 14 years of age, 2000 U.S. Census).

Whatever the strata may be, the simple random sampling method is applied within each division to achieve a sample that fairly represents each stratum. There are other sampling methods that are less common than the stratified sampling method, such as *cluster sampling, purposive sampling, snowball sampling,* and *multi stage sampling* methods. Each of the alternative sampling methods is useful in special situations, but each has limitations that may cause increased sampling error.

Types of Survey Research Designs

The instrument that is used to collect data in survey research designs is known as a *survey.* A survey is any measurement procedure that asks questions of respondents and usually takes the form of *questionnaires* or *interview instruments.* Survey instruments are designed to collect data about: (a) sociological variables, such as age, gender, social economic status, education, and occupation, or (b) psychological variables, such as opinions, attitudes, and behaviors. Surveys are conducted through regular mail, email, telephone, and face-to-face interviews.

The questionnaires used in survey research are typically mailed to participants. Questionnaires are economical to administer, and they usually allow the respondent to complete the form at their convenience. However, questionnaires have two shortcomings: (a) the response rate is often poor, and (b) they are not reliable instruments for gathering detailed responses from participants. If the response rate is poor, the sample may not represent the population, and researchers will not be able to generalize results to the population. To maximize response rates, researchers can: (a) minimize the costs for responding (time, effort, and money), (b) maximize the rewards for responding, and (c) establish trust that those rewards will be delivered.

To insure the validity of survey instruments, researchers must carefully choose the content, wording, format, and placement of questions. A successful survey requires substantial planning prior to its use. In contrast to the questionnaire format, interviews are more personal and allow the interviewer to probe for more information or ask follow-up questions. Furthermore, interviews are usually easier for the participants to complete. However, interviews are time-consuming—and interviewers must be trained. To conduct a successful interview, interviewers must motivate respondents, mitigate concerns, judge the quality of responses, and avoid interviewer biases that may threaten the validity of the participants' responses. Overall, questionnaire and interview procedures are reliable means for collecting information about a population, but great care is needed to insure their validity.

Case Examples: Survey Research in Communication Disorders.   Kritikos (2003) constructed a six-page questionnaire (25 items) to investigate speech-language pathologists' (SLP) beliefs about the language assessment of bilingual/bicultural individuals. The researcher conducted a pilot study and gathered feedback to improve the questionnaire's validity prior to its use. Questionnaires were mailed to more than 2,000 bilingual SLPs randomly selected from each of six geographic regions of the United States. The response rate was 44 percent, but 213 of the returns were incomplete so they were excluded from the analysis. Thus, a total of 811 surveys (35 percent of the total mailed) were analyzed.

Based on the survey results, Kritikos reported that many SLPs did not feel competent in assessing bilingual clients and recommended further research and education on the topic.

A second example of survey research in communication disorders utilized telephone interviews to collect data (Mirrett, Roberts, & Price, 2003). Mirrett et al. (2003) collaborated to gather information about early intervention practices and communication intervention strategies for young males with Fragile X Syndrome. The participants in the telephone interviews were 51 SLPs in North Carolina, Virginia, South Carolina, and Georgia who were referred by parents. The interview form included 22 questions and was included as an appendix in their published report. Mirrett et al. (2003) concluded their report with a discussion of limitations in their survey design, as well as clinical implications based on the results. What may have been some limitations in the research team's survey procedure? What are advantages and disadvantages for telephone interviews as a method to collect survey data? How would you describe their sample? Was it a representative sample? What was the target population? How was the researchers' ability to generalize results affected by the sampling procedure?

Replication Designs in Communication Disorders

The need to confirm or refute research results is central to the scientific approach, and *replication designs* are the means to this end. Muma (1993) explained the importance of replication to a field such as communication sciences and disorders as follows:

> Replication provides two basic kinds of information: verification or disconfirmation, both of which contribute to the substantive base of a scholarly field. Should replications yield findings similar to those in previous studies, a verification function would have been achieved. In this way the substantive base of a field achieves increased substantiation. This is very important for a field because it is well known that a single study cannot be definitive. (p. 927)

Replication designs typically aim to satisfy one or more of the following goals:

1. Establish the reliability of results.
2. Establish generality of results.
3. Establish the applicability of results to real-world situations.
4. Establish validity and generality of a concept.

The common methods for accomplishing these goals are known as: (a) conceptual replication, (b) systematic replication, and (c) direct replication.

Conceptual Replication

The conceptual replication design seeks to establish the validity and generality of particular concepts or theories. These designs are usually based on the same literature review and test the same hypothesis, but use different methods. Muma (1993) referred to these designs as *derived studies*. Conceptual replications are common designs in communication disorders research.

Systematic Replication

A second method for replication is known as *systematic replication*. Systematic replications aim to establish generalization of results to other settings or persons. Systematic replication studies ask: How robust (or fragile) is the treatment effect? To answer this question, systematic replications duplicate a previous study but also incorporate one (or two) variations in the design. For example, systematic variations are: (a) adding more subjects, (b) using different subjects, (c) using different settings, or (d) employing some other variation in the design. Systematic replication studies are small in number. Nonetheless, a number of systematic replication studies in communication disorders are reported each year. What is the value of systematic replications for evidence-based practice? What are some other possible variations of the systematic replication design?

Direct Replication

A third method for replication is known as *direct replication*. Direct replications aim to establish the reliability of previous results. To accomplish this goal, direct replication duplicates a study in every detail. The only variation is the use of new subjects. To account for the possibility of experimenter bias, direct replications are typically accomplished by independent teams of researchers. Direct replication studies are rare in communication disorders. Why are there so few direct replications of previous studies in communication disorders?

Case Examples: Replication Designs in Communication Disorders

A case example is Schlosser and Blischak's (2004) systematic replication of a previous study by the same researchers. They replicated all aspects of the earlier study but increased the number of subjects. Schlosser and Blischak (2004) described their rationale and purpose as follows:

> Because of the small number of participants, however, [the earlier] study and its explanation were deemed preliminary. The purpose of the present study, therefore, was to replicate the Schlosser et al. (1998) study with additional children in order to determine the effects of synthetic speech and print feedback on spelling acquisition and generalization by children with autism and little or no functional speech. (p. 849)

According to Schlosser and Blischak (2004), the replication study confirmed the previous results—spelling instruction with speech-generating devices was effective. Was Schlosser and Blischak's replication study an independent confirmation of results?

In another variation of the systematic replication design, Ingham, Fox, Ingham, Xiong, Zamarripa, Hardies, and Lancaster (2004) replicated an earlier study of stuttered speech. According to Ingham et al. (2004): "This article reports a gender replication study of the P. T. Fox et al. (2000) performance correlation analysis of neural systems that distinguish between normal and stuttered speech in male adults" (p. 321). In this case, the research team duplicated the details of the earlier study with one exception. They recruited females as subjects instead of males. This variation of the systematic replication design is known as *gender replication*. As a result of Ingham et al.'s (2004) the replication, the researcher team confirmed aspects of the earlier study and extended the results to females. Is there a risk of experimenter bias in the Schlosser and Blischak (2004) or Ingham et al. (2004) replications?

Conclusion: Alternative Designs in Communication Disorders Research

The breadth of opportunities for research in communication sciences and disorders is unparalleled. There are diverse topics for study—and no shortage of questions. The myriad of topics in communication disorders is matched by the diversity of research designs. There are research designs to answer virtually any question posed by clinicians and researchers. In the unusual case where there is no existing design to answer research questions, existing designs are modified or new designs invented.

According to Kerlinger, "Research designs are invented to enable the researcher to answer research questions as validly, objectively, accurately, and economically as possible" (1973, p. 301). Once the purpose and research questions are clearly articulated—the choice of a research design should be straightforward. When choosing a research design, the primary questions to ask are: (a) Does the design answer the research questions? (b) Does the design adequately test the hypothesis?

CASE STUDIES

Case 7.1   Case of Too Little Too Late

Professor Little designed a survey instrument to investigate the opinions of students currently enrolled in communication disorders programs. The survey is about research methods and the importance to clinical practice. A questionnaire was mailed to 1,000 students who were randomly selected from college programs in a national database. Two months after mailing the questionnaires, Professor Little received 101 responses. What do you see as possible shortcomings in the professor's research plan? What options are available to Professor Little?

Case 7.2   Case of the Chicken and Egg

SLPs Terrence and Mathis collected data for 10 variables related to reading performance, but they are not sure how to interpret the results. Terrence and Mathis believe that some of the variables are causally related to other variables. Their results included several statistically significant correlation coefficients with the values 0.72, 0.49, and 0.60. How should Terrence and Mathis interpret the results?

Case 7.3   Long and the Short of It

Researchers Eggers and Gomez have done extensive planning for a longitudinal study of 80-year-old men with aphasia. They expect the study to last 5 years with measurements at 1-month intervals. Eggers and Gomez have identified 22 participants and expect at least 20 to complete the study. As a consultant who specializes in research design, what problems do you foresee? What alternatives do you recommend?

Student Exercises

1. Assume that you are planning longitudinal research that will follow 20 adolescents to adulthood—a total of 8 years. What can you do to counter the potential problem of subject mortality?

2. Random selection is necessary in survey research to insure that the sample from the population is a fair sample (unbiased). How would you identify the population of kindergarten children with speech problems—and how will you select a random sample of the kindergarten children?

3. Snowball sampling was mentioned as an alternative for choosing samples from populations but not discussed. What is *snowball sampling*—and how is it employed to sample a population?

4. Locate a correlational research design in a contemporary article in a communication disorders journal. What is the independent variable? What are the dependent variables? How did the researchers explain the strength of the correlation coefficients?

5. Design a short questionnaire to survey opinions of classmates on a topic of your choice. Conduct a simple random sample of the population of students and analyze the results. Do the results represent the opinions of the population of students?

PART III

Testing Hypotheses in Communication Sciences and Disorders

8 Testing Hypotheses in Communication Disorders Research

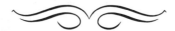

error (ĕr′ər) *n.* a mistake, the difference between a measured value and a true or theoretically correct value.

Typically, researchers seek to discover relationships between two or more variables. To this end, researchers develop hypotheses about the variables of interest prior to an experiment's beginning. *Hypotheses* are statements that describe the proposed relationship between two or more variables. Hypothesis testing is a binary decision-making process—either accepting or rejecting hypotheses based on the results of statistical tests. The goal of hypothesis testing is to use the data collected from samples to decide whether to accept or reject the hypothesis. The possibility of committing an error is important to researchers because scientific endeavors demand a high degree of reliability. For this reason, minimizing the risk of errors is critically important to the hypothesis testing process.

The Hypothesis Testing Process

Hypothesis testing begins with a statement of the hypothesis and ends with the decision to accept or reject the hypothesis. The hypothesis testing process includes six steps: (a) stating the hypothesis, (b) setting a level of risk, (c) choosing a sample size, (d) determining the critical value, (e) computing the test statistic, and (f) rejecting or accepting the hypothesis. Each step requires careful planning to ensure that the standards of scientific inquiry are met.

Step One: State the Hypothesis

Hypotheses are an integral part of the class of mathematical measurement known as *inferential statistics*. The two major classes of statistics are descriptive and inferential. Inferential statistics make conclusions about populations of individuals from sample data—whereas descriptive statistics organize, summarize, and describe the data without inferences about the populations. To illustrate, researchers might hypothesize a difference between the means of aphasic and non-aphasic adults on a test of memory skills. In doing so, researchers make suppositions about the entire population of aphasic adults. To make reliable decisions about research hypotheses, researchers consider two opposing points of view—the null hypothesis and the alternative hypothesis.

The Null Hypothesis.   To test a statistical hypothesis, what to expect when the hypothesis is true must be known. Thus, researchers hypothesize the opposite of what they expect. For example, if researchers want to demonstrate that one treatment method is more effective than another, the researchers might hypothesize that the two methods are equally effective. This is known as a *null hypothesis* (H_o) because the researchers hypothesized no difference between the two treatment methods. The null hypothesis is usually stated in terms of no relationship between variables or no difference between groups. According to Freund (1988):

> The idea of setting up a null hypothesis is common even in non-statistical thinking. It is precisely what we do in criminal proceedings, where an accused is presumed to be innocent until his guilt has been established beyond a reasonable doubt. The presumption of innocence is a null hypothesis (p. 289).

The Alternative Hypothesis.   A statement of the expected result of a research study is called the alternative hypothesis (H_A). For example, Cannito and Kondraske (1990) hypothesized that participants with spasmodic dysphonia would perform significantly slower than participants without spasmodic dysphonia on complex motor sequencing tasks. The Cannito and Kondraske hypothesis was based on their extensive review of the existing research literature. In practice, research reports typically contain one of the following: (a) a statement of the null hypothesis, (b) a statement of the alternative hypothesis, or (c) no statement of the hypothesis at all.

Step Two: Set an Acceptable Level of Risk (α)

There are four possible outcomes when testing research hypotheses: (a) the null hypothesis is accepted when it is true (correct decision), (b) the null hypothesis is rejected when it is false (correct decision), (c) the null hypothesis is rejected when in reality it is true (Type I error), or (d) the null hypothesis is accepted when in reality it is false (Type II error). The four possible outcomes are depicted in Figure 8.1.

The Decision Box in 8.1 includes two incorrect decisions known as *Type I* and *Type II errors*. The probability of a Type I error is designated by the Greek letter α (alpha). The probability of a Type II error is designated by the Greek letter β (beta). Alpha is always specified by the researcher before data collection begins. However, the value of beta cannot be determined unless the population parameters are known. Beta is seldom specified because research in communication disorders usually involves populations with unknown parameters. For example, disfluency is a common dependent variable, but its exact variation in the population is unknown. Even if beta cannot be specified, we do know that the relationship between alpha and beta is an inverse relationship. If other fac-

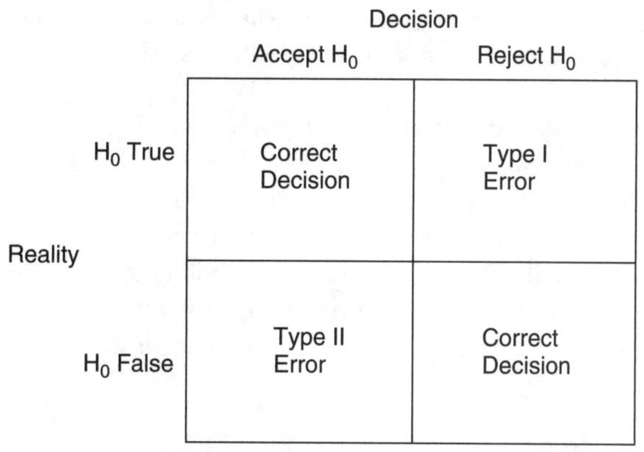

Decision

Accept H_0 Reject H_0

	Accept H_0	Reject H_0
H_0 True	Correct Decision	Type I Error
H_0 False	Type II Error	Correct Decision

Reality

Figure 8.1   Four possible outcomes when testing hypotheses.

tors are constant, an increase in alpha is accompanied by a decrease in *beta*; and a decrease in *alpha* is accompanied by an increase in beta. Rejecting a true null hypothesis (Type I error) is considered the more serious of the two possible errors. In other words, the risk of a Type I error is more serious than the risk of a Type II error. This is particularly true in medical research where rejecting a true null hypothesis (committing a Type I error) can have serious consequences for human life. Thus, alpha is conventionally set at a conservative level of .05 or less. When $\alpha = .05$, this means that the researcher is willing to risk a Type I error 5 out of 100 times. Alternatively, when $\alpha = .01$, the researcher is willing to risk a Type I error only 1 out of 100 times.

Step Three: Choose the Sample Size

The sample size (n) determines: (a) the probability distribution to be used, and (b) the power of the test. For example, the z statistic (standard normal distribution) requires relatively large samples ($n \geq 30$). However, the t *statistic* (and its distribution) is appropriate for small samples ($n < 30$) when certain assumptions are met. *Power* is defined as the probability of rejecting the null hypothesis when it is false—a correct decision. Sample size is one of several factors that influence the power of a statistical test. A larger sample usually results in a more powerful test of the null hypothesis. The conclusions drawn from studies with small samples such as $n < 10$ are a high risk for accepting the null hypothesis when it is false (Type II error).

Step Four: Determine the Critical Value

Statistical hypothesis testing requires a cut-off point that can be used to separate sample results that should lead to rejecting H_0 from sample results that should lead to accepting H_0. This cut-off point is known as the *critical value*. Critical values are found by using tables for either the standard normal distribution or *Student's t distribution*. The critical value depends on: (a) *alpha*—the level at which the researcher agrees to accept or reject H_o, and (b) the alternative hypothesis (H_A).

Two Types of Alternative Hypotheses.   There are two types of alternative hypotheses: (a) *one-tailed* (directional) and (b) *two-tailed* (nondirectional) hypotheses. A one-tailed hypothesis predicts the direction of results. For example, a researcher might hypothesize that treatment A is better than treatment B. This is a directional hypothesis. In contrast, a two-tailed hypothesis does not predict the direction of results. For example, a researcher might hypothesize that treatment A is different than treatment B but not predict which treatment is better. The sampling distribution for a one-tailed hypothesis test is pictured in Figure 8.2.

The Rejection Region.   The shaded area in Figure 8.2 extends from the cut-off point (*critical value*) and divides the distribution into two regions. The area to the left of the shaded area is the rejection region while the shaded area is the acceptance region.

The rejection region may be located in either tail depending on the direction specified by the alternative hypothesis. If the expected result is a positive difference, the rejection region is located in the right tail. If the expected result is a negative difference, the rejection region is located in the left tail. When the test statistic—otherwise known as the *observed value*—is less than the critical value, the null hypothesis is rejected. When the test statistic is greater than the critical value, the null hypothesis is accepted. A *two-tailed hypothesis test* is pictured in Figure 8.3.

The two-tailed hypothesis test divides the rejection region equally between the two ends of the distribution. If other factors are constant, a one-tailed test is more powerful than a two-tailed test because the rejection region is larger—concentrated on one end of the sampling distribution. A two-tailed test divides the rejection region in halves—half in each tail. Thus, in the case of a two-tailed test, the probability of rejecting the null hypothesis is reduced.

In the case of the z statistic, the critical value is a standard score. For example, if α = .05 and H_A is one-tailed, the critical value is -1.645 (1.645 standard deviation units below the population mean). If α = .05 and H_A is two-tailed, the critical value is ± 1.96—almost two standard deviation units above or below the population mean. It is easier to reject the null hypothesis with a one-tailed test. Thus, a one-tailed test is more powerful. However, the use of one-tailed alternative hypotheses has been criticized for the fol-

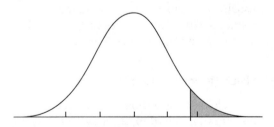

Figure 8.2 Sampling distribution for a one-tailed (directional) hypothesis test.

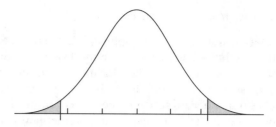

Figure 8.3   Sampling distribution for a two-tailed (nondirectional) hypothesis test.

lowing reasons: (a) a one-tailed test ignores the possibility of an unexpected difference in the opposite direction; (b) a one-tailed test is more vulnerable to error if a distribution is not normal; and (c) a one-tailed test might be selected when a two-tailed test is more appropriate.

Several guidelines are useful for planning research as well as for evaluating research reports. First, hypotheses should be two tailed unless there is compelling evidence that the expected result will be directional. Second, the choice of directional or non-directional hypotheses should be decided before a study begins. Finally, researchers should provide a sound rationale when electing one-tailed hypotheses. An illustration is Yoder's (1989) study where one-tailed hypothesis tests were elected, and Yoder explained that one-tailed tests were justified because the purpose was to replicate the results of an earlier study by confirming a relationship between maternal speech and children's language learning.

Step Five: Compute the Test Statistic

The *test statistic* is a standard score such as z or a t statistic. These scores indicate the number of standard errors the sample statistic is from the hypothesized parameter. The general formula for a test statistic (observed value) is given in Figure 8.4.

Choosing a Test Statistic.   The choice of a test statistic depends on several factors: (a) the hypothesis, (b) the distribution of the target population, (c) sample size, and (d) other sample characteristics. For example, if researchers hypothesize a difference between two sample means, the t statistic is an appropriate test statistic. However, if the population is not normally distributed, a *nonparametric* (distribution free) statistic may be more appropriate. Nonparametric tests are a special class of inferential statistics that do not depend on the population conforming to a prescribed shape because the raw data are replaced by their ranks. A common nonparametric test is the *Mann-Whitney U test* (also known as the *Wilcoxon rank sum test*)—but there are nonparametric tests to fit most experimental designs.

$$\text{Test Statistic} = \frac{(\text{statistic}) - (\text{parameter})}{\text{standard error of the statistic}}$$

Figure 8.4   Compute the Test Statistic.

Step Six: Make a Decision about H_o

After the test statistic is computed, it is compared to the critical value. If the test statistic's absolute value exceeds the critical value, the null hypothesis is rejected. If the test statistic does not exceed the critical value, the null hypothesis is accepted. If the null hypothesis is rejected, the alternative hypothesis is supported but not proven. Kerlinger (1979) described research outcomes as continually better approximations of the *truth* but never attaining complete truth. Furthermore, a result may be statistically significant but not of any practical value because statistical significance alone indicates the reliability of accepting a research hypothesis but not the importance of the result. In practice, clinicians are concerned with clinical relevance, and a statistically significant result may not be clinically relevant. Clinical significance is determined by several factors, and one of those factors is *effect size*—an indicator of practical significance. The notion of practical significance is important to establishing evidence-based clinical practices (cf. Meline & Paradiso, 2003).

The Normal Distribution

Many variables in communication disorders are continuously distributed as opposed to being placed into discrete categories. A *distribution* is simply a pattern of scores. The distribution of a variable provides information about individual cases as well as information about the group of scores. The distributions for categorical variables are displayed in bar graphs, whereas the distributions for continuous variables are usually displayed in line graphs or histograms. The normal distribution is the most important one of many statistical distributions. The normal distribution is a theoretical distribution based on the general equation developed by the French mathematician, De Moivre (1667–1754). It provides a model for evaluating the distributions of many real-life variables. Normal distributions are useful for determining the probability of certain outcomes. De Moivre developed the general equation by observing games of chance, for example, a coin flip produces two possible outcomes—heads or tails. Each possibility has an equal chance of occurring. The probability of tails is 1/2—one possibility of tails divided by two possi-

---

Technology Note

The normal distribution is also known as the *Gaussian distribution* because Carl Friedrich Gauss was one of the first to use the distribution when he analyzed astronomical data in 1809, but Abraham De Moivre [*du mwA' vru*] is credited with the discovery circa 1733. De Moivre developed the theoretical distribution years before Gauss was born—but his paper was not discovered until 1924 by Karl Pearson. De Moivre also pioneered the theory of probability in *The Doctrine of Change* published in 1718. Born in Paris, Abraham De Moivre tutored mathematics for a living but died in poverty in 1754.

ble outcomes. If enough coins are flipped, the distribution of outcomes should approximate De Moivre's normal distribution—half the outcomes will be tails and half will be heads. However, some of the coins in the sample will not be fair. In other words, an individual coin may land heads 6 out of 10 flips. Another coin may favor tails. Nonetheless, the pattern of outcomes for all the coins in the sample will approximate a normal distribution with a bell shape as pictured in Figure 8.5.

The normal distribution has three important characteristics:

1. The normal distribution is unimodal (one mode at the center) and symmetrical (the right half mirrors the left half—as opposed to a bimodal distribution which has two modes.
2. The normal distribution is continuous.
3. The normal distribution is asymptotic—the curved line gets closer to the horizontal axis as it moves away from the center but does not touch the axis.

Because different variables have different means and standard deviations, an infinite number of distributions are possible. Although all of these distributions may approximate De Moivre's model, they are not comparable because of their different units of measurement. This problem is resolved by transforming all normal distributions to fit the standard normal distribution.

The Standard Normal Distribution

The standard normal distribution is a useful tool for describing a normally distributed variable. The notion behind the standard normal distribution is that all normal distributions can be converted to a common distribution with the same mean and standard deviation—a mean of zero and a standard deviation of one. The standard normal distribution is pictured in Figure 8.6.

Because the standard normal distribution has a prescribed mean and standard deviation, the proportion of scores in a given area under the bell-shaped curve is always the same. Thus, the area between −1 and +1 standard deviations always includes 68 percent

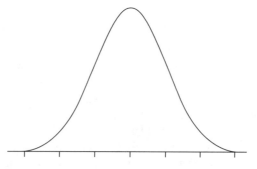

Figure 8.5 The normal distribution—a bell-shaped curve.

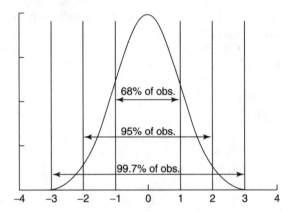

Figure 8.6   The standard normal distribution.

of the total distribution of scores. Likewise, the area between −2 and +2 standard deviations includes 95 percent of the scores—and the area between −3 and +3 standard deviations includes 99 percent of the scores. This information is important for determining the probability of an outcome. For example, the likelihood of a score falling ±2 or greater standard deviations from the mean is 5 percent—5 times out of 100.

Standard Units

A single score in the distribution of scores can be represented by a standard unit of measure known as a *z score*. A z score—also known as a standard score—is derived from the equation below.

$$z = \frac{X - \overline{X}}{S}$$

z = the standard value
x = any one score
$\overline{X}$ = the mean of the sample distribution
S = the standard deviation of the sample distribution

The z score is a measure of individual location. In other words, it tells us where individual scores are located within a distribution of scores. The z score tells us how many standard deviations the corresponding value of *x* lies above or below the mean. By adopting a standard unit of measure such as the z score, we can make comparisons between different variables are possible. For example, if a 5-year-old child obtains a raw score of 59 on the *Test for Auditory Comprehension of Language-3* (Carrow-Woolfolk, 1999) and a score of 60 on the *Peabody Picture Vocabulary Test-III* (Dunn & Dunn, 1997), a comparison between scores is not meaningful because the test distributions are different. However, a clinician can compare the z scores from the two different assessments with the equivalent standard scores: −1.00 (TACL-3) and 0.00 (PPVT-III). In this example,

Technology Note

Microsoft Excel's NORMDIST function returns the normal distribution for a selected mean and standard deviation. If the mean is 0 and standard deviation is 1, NORMDIST returns the standard normal distribution. The Excel function NORMSDIST returns the standard normal distribution and the area under the normal curve for a given z score. NORMSDIST can be used in place of a table of standard normal curve areas. For example, a z score of +0.67 returns an area of 75 percent which is the proportion of scores that fall below the z score. A z score of −0.67 returns 25 percent—the proportion of scores below −0.67. The area between −0.67 and +0.67 is 50 percent.

the TACL-3 score is one standard deviation lower than the PPVT-III score—a significant clinical finding.

A table of values known as a *standard normal distribution table* is displayed in Table 8.1. It contains z scores from 0.0 to 3.0 and proportions for the areas between means and z *scores*. For example, the proportion of the area between the mean and a z score equal to 1.5 is 0.4332 (43 percent). Because the distribution is symmetrical, the area between the mean and $z = +1.5$ is the same as the area between the mean and $z = -1.5$. Thus, the proportion of the area between −1.5 and +1.5 equals 86 percent.

Table 8.1   Areas Under the Standard Normal Curve.

z	Area between the mean and z	z	Area between the mean and z
0.0	.0000	1.6	.4452
0.1	.0398	1.7	.4554
0.2	.0793	1.8	.4641
0.3	.1179	1.9	.4713
0.4	.1554	2.0	.4772
0.5	.1915	2.1	.4821
0.6	.2257	2.2	.4861
0.7	.2580	2.3	.4893
0.8	.2881	2.4	.4918
0.9	.3159	2.5	.4938
1.0	.3413	2.6	.4953
1.1	.3643	2.7	.4965
1.2	.3849	2.8	.4974
1.3	.4032	2.9	.4981
1.4	.4192	3.0	.4987
1.5	.4332		

Transformed Standard Scores

Because z scores include negative values and decimals, they are somewhat difficult to report and may be misleading to clients, parents, and others. For this reason, z scores are often transformed into a distribution of standard scores with a mean of 100 and a standard deviation equal to 15 units. The transformation is accomplished by multiplying each z score by 15 and adding 100 as indicated in this formula.

$$\text{Transformed score} = (15)\,(z) + 100$$

As a clinical example, the *Peabody Picture Vocabulary Test-III* (1997) includes *standard score equivalents—transformed standard scores—*with a mean of 100 and a standard deviation of 15. The use of standard scores simplifies the interpretation of the scores. The mean is 100 and the standard deviation is 15, but the choice of values for the mean and standard deviation is an arbitrary one.

Shapes of Frequency Distributions

Data can be distributed in a variety of ways, taking on almost any shape or form. However, most frequency distributions can be described by a small number of standard shapes. The most important of these standard distributions is the bell-shaped normal distribution. However, even if a variable is normally distributed in the population, a sample of the population is not always normally distributed. Thus, other shapes are needed to describe distributions that are not normally distributed.

Skewed Distributions

One class of frequency distributions that is not bell-shaped is known as *skewed distributions*. Skewed distributions are not symmetrical. For example, a negatively skewed distribution is pictured in Figure 8.7. *Skewness* is an indicator of symmetry—or a lack of symmetry.

A graph is informative because it provides a picture of the degree of skewness. A negatively skewed distribution has more scores with larger values toward the right tail, whereas a positively skewed distribution has more scores with larger values toward the left tail. A positive skew is pictured in Figure 8.8.

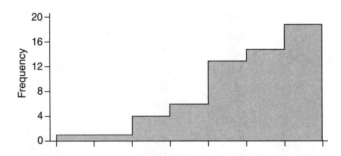

Figure 8.7   A negatively skewed distribution of scores.

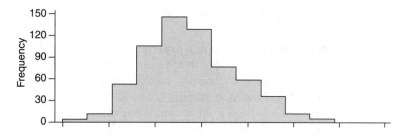

Figure 8.8 A positively skewed distribution of scores.

Other Common Shapes for Frequency Distributions

Symmetrical distributions including the normal distribution are characterized by their kurtosis. *Kurtosis* is a measure of peakedness. It measures how fat or thin the tails of a distribution are relative to a normal distribution. A *mesokurtic distribution,* such as the normal curve, is characterized by a moderate degree of peakedness. If a large proportion of scores is located at the center of the distribution, the distribution is described as *leptokurtic.* The upper figure in Figure 8.9 is leptokurtic, and the lower figure is a *platykurtic distribution.* Platykurtic distributions are characterized by a large proportion of scores in the tails.

If research requires a precise measure of kurtosis, it is computed as a coefficient of skewness. The *Pearsonian coefficient of skewness* (SK) is a simple statistic for comparing a distribution's mean and median to measure skewness. The formula for SK is displayed below. If a distribution is perfectly symmetrical, the value of SK will equal zero. The distribution of scores becomes more skewed as SK approaches $\pm$ 3.00.

$$SK = \frac{3(\text{mean} - \text{median})}{\text{standard deviation}}$$

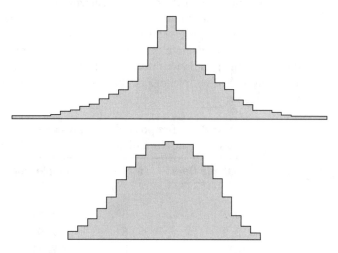

Figure 8.9 Leptokurtic and platykurtic distribution shapes.

The Distribution of a Sample Statistic

A distribution is defined as a pattern of scores. All variables have distributions. For example, height is a variable that is distributed in the population from low to high. Statistics such as the mean, median, and standard deviation have distributions as well. The distribution of a sample statistic is a basic concept underlying statistical inference. The sample selected from a population is one of many possible samples. Thus, the statistic, which is calculated from the sample, is only one of many possible statistics. The distribution of a sample statistic tells us how often different values of that statistic should occur if samples of the same size are collected over and over from the same population. One example of the distribution of a sample statistic is known as the *distribution of sample means*.

The Distribution of Sample Means

As an example, consider a population with five cases ($N = 5$) and the scores [3, 5, 7, 9, 11]. Calculations of the population mean (μ) and standard deviation (σ) are accomplished here:

$$\mu = \frac{3 + 5 + 7 + 9 + 11}{5} = 7$$

$$\sigma = \sqrt{\frac{(3 - 7)^2 + (5 - 7)^2 + (7 - 7)^2 + (9 - 7)^2 + (11 - 7)^2}{5}} = 2.83$$

Given the population of $N = 5$, there are 10 possible random samples of size $n = 2$ that can be drawn from the population. The ten samples and their means are listed in Table 8.2. The distribution of sample means from the example is displayed in Table 8.2. Distributions such as in Figure 8.10 are known as *probability distributions* because they provide information about the chance occurrence of a particular outcome.

A distribution of sample means is used to answer questions such as: How often will a mean IQ of 80 be observed with a sample of 30 cases if the mean IQ in the population is 100? Given the example, what is the chance of observing a mean of 10 with a sample size $n = 2$ if the population mean is 7? Because the number 10 only occurs once in the distribution of 10 sample means, the answer is 0.10 (10 percent). What is the chance of

Table 8.2   Ten possible samples and sample means drawn from a population of size $N = 5$.

Sample Data	Means	Sample Data	Means
3, 5	4	5, 9	7
3, 7	5	5, 11	8
3, 9	6	7, 9	8
3, 11	7	7, 11	9
5, 7	6	9, 11	10

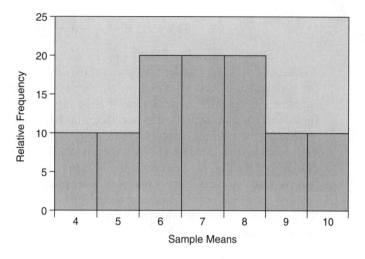

Figure 8.10   Distribution of sample means for a population of size $N = 5$.

the sample mean differing from the population mean by more than 1? The answer is 40 percent because 4 of the 10 sample means differ from the population mean by more than 1. It is fairly easy to compute probabilities when the distribution of sample means is known. However, it is usually not practical to construct a distribution of sample means because the target population is too large and the number of sample means is unwieldy.

The Standard Error of the Mean

It is not practical to collect all possible samples and then construct a distribution of sample means to determine the variation of a sample mean from the population mean. However, the necessary information is derived from two theorems that express essential facts about distributions of sample means. The first of the two theorems states: (a) the mean of the distribution of sample means equals the population mean, and (b) the distribution of sample means is less variable than the population. In the example, the population mean equaled seven. The mean of the sample means is calculated:

$$\mu_x = \frac{4 + 5 + 6 + 6 + 7 + 7 + 8 + 8 + 9 + 10}{10} = 7$$

Thus, the supposition that the mean of the sample means (μ_x) equals the population mean is supported ($\mu_x = \mu$). The second part of the theorem says that the standard deviation of the sample means is smaller than the standard deviation of the population. The standard deviation of the sample means is known as the *standard error of the mean*, abbreviated as S.E.M.

$$Exact\ S.E.M. = \frac{\sigma}{\sqrt{n}}\ or\ \frac{\sigma}{\sqrt{n}}x\sqrt{\frac{N-n}{N-1}}$$

To calculate the exact standard deviation of the sample means, the standard deviation of the population (σ) is needed and the number of cases in the sample (n). The left most equation expresses the necessary calculation for populations of infinite size—and the right most equation adds a correction factor for finite populations of size N.

Because the example involves a finite population ($N = 5$), the second of the two formulas shown in the formula above is appropriate. The standard error of the mean is calculated as 1.73. The standard deviation of the population is 2.83. Thus the proposition that the distribution of sample means is less variable than the population is supported ($\sigma_x < \sigma$). However, speech-language pathologists and audiologists usually do not know the population parameters for the variables of interest. Fortunately, the second of the two theorems—the *central limit theorem*—provides a solution.

The Central Limit Theorem

The central limit theorem (CLT) proposed that the distribution of sample means will be approximately normal if the sample is large enough. Even if a variable is not normally distributed in the population, the sampling distribution will be approximately normal with a large sample. A sample of size $n \geq 30$ is generally regarded as sufficiently large. Computer simulations involving large sets of data and many sample means are used for demonstrating the validity of the central limit theorem. In fact, Norušis (1988) has proven by computer simulation that even a uniform distribution has a distribution of sample means that approximates a normal distribution. Thus, the central limit theorem justifies the use of normal-curve methods for solving many statistical problems. It does not matter if the variable of interest is normally distributed in the population because the means calculated from samples will be normally distributed anyway. On the other hand, if the variable is normally distributed in the population—the distribution of sample means will be normal for samples of any size.

Estimating Population Parameters

If the characteristics of a target population are unknown, the population parameters can be estimated from sample characteristics. This is possible because the central limit theorem says that a sampling distribution of sufficient size is approximately normal. Thus, the standard error of the mean is estimated from the standard deviation of the sample as follows:

$$Estimated\ S.E.M. = \frac{SD}{\sqrt{n}}$$

Point Estimates vs. Interval Estimates

A single number derived from a sample and used to estimate a population value is called a point estimate. In the case of the formula above, the point estimator is the standard deviation (SD) of the sample. However, point estimates present a problem. A sample statistic reflects the population parameter but also contains sampling error. The sampling error is the difference between the population value and the sample value. Thus, calculations based on point estimates are not exactly correct. Sampling error cannot be eliminated, but it can be managed by using another kind of estimation known as *interval estimation*. Interval estimation builds on point estimates to establish a range of values that we can say with some confidence contains the population parameter. This range of values is known as a *confidence interval* (CI). The general equation for constructing confidence intervals is as follows:

$$CI = statistic \pm (critical\ value)\ (S.E.\ statistic)$$

To construct a confidence interval for the population mean, a critical value is chosen. Because the distribution of sample means is assumed to be normally distributed, 95 percent of the sample means are expected to fall within ± 2 standard errors of the population mean. Thus, the critical value equals 2 for a 95 percent confidence interval. The critical value will depend on the level of confidence chosen by the researcher. For example, a 90 percent confidence interval requires a critical value of 1.65. The lower limit of the CI is calculated by subtracting two standard errors from the estimated mean. The upper limit of the CI is determined by adding two standard errors to the estimated mean. For example, if the sample mean is 8 and SEM equals 1.5, the 95 percent confidence interval is as follows:

$$CI_{95} = 8 \pm (2)\ (1.5) = 6.5\ to\ 9.5$$

In this case, the interval is expected to contain the true population mean 95 out of 100 times.

Student's t Distributions

For samples of size $n = 30$ and larger, the distribution of a sample statistic can be assumed to be normal. However, samples smaller than 30 present a problem. Fortunately, an alternative distribution is available for small samples. William Gossett, a young chemist who worked on quality control at a brewery in Dublin, made an important discovery circa 1900. Gossett found that, in the case of small samples, the sampling distributions were substantially different from the normal distribution. Gossett also noted that the sampling distributions increasingly approximated the normal distribution as the sample size increased. From these observations, Gossett derived a family of distributions, which change as sample size changes. To ensure his anonymity, Gossett published his results in 1908 under the pseudonym "Student." Thus, this family of distributions came to be known as *Student's t distributions*. Like the normal distribution, Student's t distributions are symmetrical, bell-shaped, and centered on the mean—but the distributions change as sample sizes change. Because research in communication disorders may involve small samples ($n < 30$), researchers often depend on Student's t distributions to test hypotheses.

Conclusion: Testing Hypotheses in Communication Disorders Research

An important research goal is discovery of relationships between two or more variables. Prior to beginning an experiment, researchers develop hypotheses about the variables to be studied. The hypothesis testing process includes six steps: (a) stating the hypothesis, (b) setting a level of risk, (c) choosing a sample size, (d) determining the critical value, (e) computing the test statistic, and (f) rejecting or accepting the hypothesis. Each step is equally important, and each step requires careful planning to achieve the highest standards of scientific inquiry.

CASE STUDIES

Case 8.1   Adam's Dilemma

Adam is planning a student research project, but he is in a quandary about choosing the direction for the research hypothesis. Adam plans to investigate a hypothesized relationship between vocal tremor (the dependent variable) and chronological age (the independent variable). As a colleague and fellow student, what is your advice to Adam?

Case 8.2   Clinical Case for Priscilla

Priscilla's clinical supervisor, Dolores Goodbody, assigned a preschool child to Priscilla for a comprehensive evaluation. After completing the evaluation, Priscilla was asked to chart a comparison of outcomes for three standardized test instruments—all designed to measure development of speech and language skills. The problem is that each of the three tests reports results in different units of measurement. How can Priscilla compare the outcomes for the three different test instruments?

Case 8.3   Question of Parameters

Steven is planning a senior thesis—a comparative study of two groups of four children as participants. He is anticipating an analysis of the data with the help of inferential statistical procedures. Steve's first choice for a statistical analysis is the t test procedure. As a consultant, what is your best advice for Steven?

Student Exercises

1. Search the current volume of the *Journal of Speech-Language-Hearing Research* for a quantitative research report. What is the hypothesis? Is it stated as the null or alternative hypothesis? Is the hypothesis directional or non-directional?

2. Identify a contemporary research report and evaluate the authors' steps for testing the hypothesis. Evaluate how the researchers accomplished each of the six steps in the hypothesis testing process.

3. Computer applications are an important asset for research data analysis. Acquaint yourself with Microsoft Excel's NORMDIST function and generate the standard normal distribution using NORMDIST.

4. Find a contemporary research report that utilizes distribution-free inferential statistics in its analysis of data section. Why did the researchers choose a nonparametric statistic? Do you think that their choice of a nonparametric statistic was justified?

5. Search the current reports of research for a table of data from the measurement of a variable. Calculate the means, the median, the standard deviation, and the Pearsonian coefficient of skewness (SK). Evaluate the distribution of scores for skewness.

CHAPTER

9

Quantitative Analysis in Communication Disorders Research

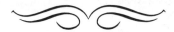

analyze (ân′ə-līz′) *v.* to examine, investigate, interpret; resolve problems by reducing the conditions in them to equations; to study the exact relations existing between quantities or magnitudes.

The purpose of most experiments is to test one or more hypotheses concerning some characteristics (parameters) of the population. For example, Reynolds, Callihan, and Browning (2003) tested the hypothesis: "children between the ages of 37 and 54 months who participate in lessons designed to teach them to identify and produce rhyming words [will] make greater gains in their awareness of rhyme than will a similar group of children who do not receive this training" (p 42). What did the research team predict as an experimental outcome? What might have been their reason for predicting the outcome in one direction? The participants in the Reynolds et al. (2003) study were 16 children (10 males, 6 females) enrolled in a local daycare center. What population was targeted by the Reynolds et al. team? What characteristics of the population were tested?

To test hypotheses about populations, quantitative researchers choose analytical procedures that match the design of their studies. For example, a pretest-posttest design usually involves two observations of the same subjects—one observation before treatment and one observation after treatment. Thus, a statistical test that matches the pretest-posttest design is a test for differences between two conditions, also known as a *related-samples test* because the same subjects are observed both before and after treatment.

The selection of analytical procedures for testing hypotheses depends on the level of measurement for the dependent variable—nominal, ordinal, interval, or ratio—as well as the experimental design. The majority of quantitative analyses in communication disorders research are performed with either t-test or analysis of variance (ANOVA) procedures. Both t test and analysis of variance statistical procedures require continuous data, usually interval level of measurement. A statistical procedure for analyzing categorical

Technology Note

Many statistical software packages are available for analyzing quantitative data on desktop computers. The most commonly used statistical software packages are SPSS, SYSTAT, and MINITAB. Each is available for both Windows and Macintosh operating systems, and each is menu driven making them user friendly and relatively easy to learn. SYSTAT and SPSS are general-purpose statistical packages that offer a variety of data manipulations, statistical analyses, and graphing tools. Minitab is a basic statistics and graphics package that is often used for student instruction in introductory statistics courses. The current version of Minitab is Release 14, and it includes basic statistics, multivariate analysis, nonparametrics, graphics and more: *http://www.minitab.com*. The current SPSS package is version 13.0: *http://www.spss.com*. The current SYSTAT package is version 11: *http://www.systat.com*. SPSS and SYSTAT include descriptive statistics, correlation, re-sampling, regression, inferential statistics, factor analysis, graphing, and more.

(nominal level) data—and often employed in communication disorders research—is the chi-square (X^2) test. The *chi-square test* is a popular statistical procedure because it is simple to calculate and easily interpreted.

There are many different experimental designs (simple to complex) and a variety of t test, analysis of variance, and chi-square procedures to match. The results of t test and analysis of variance procedures are known as *inferential statistics* because they purport to infer something about the population. The use of inferential statistical procedures such as t test and analysis of variance presumes that samples are randomly selected from the population. *Random sampling* implies that each member of the population has an equal chance of being selected. If samples are not randomly selected, an experiment's conclusions are limited. In the case of Reynolds et al. (2003), the research team selected 16 children enrolled in a local daycare center as participants for a study of rhyme. Did they employ random sampling to select participants? Were the Reynolds et al. (2003) conclusions limited in scope?

The chi-square test—also known as the *test of independence*—is a widely used nonparametric statistical procedure. The chi-square test relies on weaker, less accurate data for input than do t test and analysis of variance procedures; consequently the outcome is less reliable. Nonetheless, the t test, analysis of variance, and chi-square tests are useful statistical procedures for the analysis of data in communication disorders when properly used. The results of t tests, analyses of variance, and chi-square tests are typically found in the *Results* section of research reports. Authors do not always describe their statistical procedures in detail, but informed consumers are usually able to evaluate the procedures and results based on the available information. The majority of research in communication disorders utilizes: (a) tests for differences between two groups or conditions, (b) tests for differences between multiple groups or conditions, or (c) tests for analyzing categorical data.

Tests for Differences Between Two Groups or Conditions

Many research questions in communication disorders (especially questions pertaining to clinical efficacy) are appropriately investigated by testing for differences between two groups, or two conditions within one group. For example, a question about the efficacy of a specific therapy technique might be tested by randomly assigning subjects to experimental and control groups, wherein the experimental group receives the therapy, and the control group receives a salutary treatment or no treatment at all. In this case, the *observed outcome* is the difference between the two groups (experimental vs. control); usually the difference is between means. If the difference between the two groups is nil or too small to be significant, researchers may conclude that the proposed therapy is not likely to be effective in clinical practice. However, if the difference between the two groups is large enough to be significant and the experimental group benefits from the treatment, researchers may conclude that the therapy is likely to be effective in clinical practice.

Research designs that employ two groups of subjects as participants are known as *unrelated-measures designs* because the two samples (experimental and control groups) are composed of different subjects. It is also known as a *between-subjects design* because the comparison is between two groups of subjects. An alternative to the between-subjects design is the *pretest-posttest design,* which is a popular research design in communication disorders, in part because of its similarity to the clinical model. In this case, a baseline measurement is established during the pretest stage, an experimental treatment is introduced in the second stage, and a posttest measurement is performed in the final (outcome) stage. If the posttest measurement of the dependent variable exceeds the pretest measurement, researchers may conclude that the intervening treatment was responsible for the change. Research designs that employ pretest-posttest observations with an intervening treatment are known as *related-measures designs* because the two samples (pretest and posttest) are composed of the same subjects.

The related-measures design is also known as a *within-subjects design* because the comparison is between two or more conditions within the same group of subjects.

The statistical procedures for testing differences between two groups of subjects or, alternatively, between two conditions within the same group of subjects are classified as either: (a) tests for unrelated samples, or (b) tests for related samples. The choice of one statistical test or the other depends on the research design. Two-group designs typically require statistical tests for unrelated samples, and pretest-posttest designs require statistical tests for related samples.

Tests for Unrelated Samples

The most popular statistical procedure for testing differences between two groups of subjects in communication disorders is Student's t test. Student's t test was devised by Gossett in the early 1900s, and he published the work under the pseudonym *Student.* Gossett's work was a solution to the problem of small samples (n < 30). Gossett devised distributions of scores based on *degrees of freedom,* and as the degrees of freedom increased in number, the distributions approximated a normal distribution of scores. For small samples, the t distribution is typically bell-shaped but narrower than the normal distribution (*leptokurtic*). For samples of 30 or more observations, the t distribution approximates the normal distribution of scores. The t test is especially designed for testing hypotheses based on small samples (n < 30). If the sample size is large (n ≥ 30), z (normal standard deviation) is an appropriate test for differences between two groups. The z test is based on the normal distribution of scores, otherwise known as the *normal curve*. The proportions of area under the normal curve are found in the appendix of most basic statistics books.

The outcome of Student's t-test procedure is known as the *t ratio*. The t ratio is the ratio of the difference between the means of the two groups of subjects divided by the *standard error of the difference (S.E.D.)* as shown in the following formula:

$$\text{Student's } t = \frac{mean_1 - mean_2}{S.E.D.}$$

S.E.D. is a measure of the variability or dispersion of the scores attributable to error. In the case of *unrelated (independent) samples*, the standard error of the difference is estimated from the square root of the pooled variances for the two groups as indicated below:

$$\text{S.E.D.}_{\text{unrelated samples}} = \sqrt{S_1^2/N_1} + S_2^2/N_2$$

$$\text{degrees of freedom} = N_1 + N_2 - 2$$

The t test for *unrelated samples* is appropriate for answering the question: Is an observed difference between two groups of subjects attributable to chance? If the answer is *no,* the alternative hypothesis is accepted. The t test for unrelated samples is sometimes used in communication disorders to test the equivalency (or non-equivalency) of two groups of subjects. For example, Reynolds et al. (2003) randomly assigned 16 children to experimental and control groups. However, the children in the control group were slightly older (mean = 46 months; SD = 6.5) than children in the experimental group (mean = 42.4 months; SD = 5.1)—a difference of 3.6 months. Because *group equivalency* was an important consideration for the Reynolds et al. (2003) research team, they asked the question: Is the difference between mean ages for the experimental and control groups a significant one? To test the hypothesis that the difference was not significant, the researchers employed a t test for unrelated samples. The result was not significant, p > .05. The .05 (5 percent) level of confidence is the conventional cut-off point for accepting or rejecting the null hypothesis in communication disorders research. If p = .05, the probability is that 5 times out of 100 you would find a statistically significant difference between means (by chance) even if there was none. The .05 level is considered a tolerable level of risk, but anything greater than .05 is considered unacceptable.

The 95 percent confidence interval for the Reynolds et al. (2003) difference between means is: CI (95 percent) = −9.33 < difference < 2.13. *Confidence intervals* are statistical procedures for establishing the precision of a result, as well as deciding whether to accept or reject the null hypothesis. If the confidence interval contains zero, the null hypothesis is accepted. The width of the confidence interval indicates the precision of measurement, and precision is directly related to sample size. In the Reynolds et al. (2003) case, the small sample (n = 16) produced a relatively wide confidence interval.

Does the confidence interval for the Reynolds et al. (2003) difference between means include zero? How should this result be interpreted?

Reynolds et al. (2003) used random assignment to constitute experimental and control groups. Nonetheless, the two groups differed in chronological age by 3.5 months—a statistically nonsignificant difference. Why did the two groups differ by 3.5 months of age? If the study is replicated, how might you achieve a smaller difference in chronological age between experimental and control groups?

To correctly use the t test with unrelated samples, several assumptions are necessary. First, subjects must be randomly and independently sampled. Second is the assumption that the two groups are independent and unrelated. If the assumption of independent samples is not met, alternative procedures must be used. Third, the distribution of differences between means must be normally distributed. This is not a problem when sample size is ≥ 30 but may be problematic for smaller samples. Researchers typically inspect the pattern of the data for its distributional characteristics.

If a distribution of scores is not symmetrical, researchers may choose to transform the data to achieve a more normal distribution. *Transformations* are single mathematical operations—such as square, square root, reciprocal, and log functions—that are applied to the data and replace each of the original data values. A drawback to transforming data is that it changes the metric (unit of measure) in which the data are analyzed. As a consequence, the results may be more difficult to interpret.

The fourth assumption that applies to the t test for unrelated samples requires the two groups to have equal (or near equal) variances—known as *homogeneity of variance*. The F statistic (displayed below) is a simple test for homogeneity of variances.

$$F \text{ statistic} = \frac{SD_1}{SD_2}$$

degrees of freedom $= n_1 - 1$ (numerator), $n_2 - 1$ (denominator)

Technology Note

The choice of parametric statistics carries the burden of meeting certain assumptions to ensure a valid test—(a) normality of sample distributions, and (b) homogeneity of sample variances. The simplest method to evaluate normality is to visualize the frequency distribution histogram. A second method is to examine the values of skewness and kurtosis for sample distributions. Microsoft Excel includes the histogram function in Tools/Data Analysis menus and includes KURT and SKEW functions in the statistical functions menu. Statistical applications such as MINITAB and SPSS include similar functions. A third method for testing normality is the *Kolmogorov-Smirnov Test* included in MINITAB and SPSS applications (alternatives are *Anderson-Darling* and *Ryan-Joiner tests*). Tests for homogeneity of variance include the F-test for two samples and *Bartlett's and Levene's tests* for multiple samples. These tests are included in many statistical software applications.

Its application is straightforward. The computation of F includes the standard deviations (SD) for the two samples. For example, Reynolds et al. (2003) randomly assigned 16 subjects to two groups, but variance for chronological age was greater in the control group ($SD = 6.5$) versus the experimental group ($SD = 5.1$). To test for homogeneity of variances, the larger value is entered into the numerator and the smaller value in the denominator as follows:

$$F \text{ statistic} = \frac{6.5}{5.1} = 1.27$$

$$\text{degrees of freedom} = 7 \text{ (numerator)}, 7 \text{ (denominator)}$$

To evaluate the result, the observed value (1.27) is compared to the critical value derived from a *Table of Critical Values* for the F Distribution (found in the appendix of most basic statistics books). The *Table of Critical Values* is entered with the degrees of freedom associated with the F ratio's numerator and denominator. In the Reynolds et al. (2003) case, the critical value for F equals 6.99. If the observed value equals or exceeds the critical value, the null hypothesis is rejected. In this case, 1.27 (observed value) is less than 6.99 (critical value), so the null hypothesis is accepted. Thus, the variances for experimental and control groups in the Reynolds et al. (2003) study can be assumed to be homogeneous.

If assumptions of normality or equal variances cannot otherwise be met, an alternative for testing differences between means is *nonparametric* procedures—also known as distribution-free tests. The *Mann-Whitney U test* is a nonparametric statistical procedure for cases of two unrelated samples. Nonparametric tests are typically applied to ordinal data (e.g., ranks) and are not dependent on the usual assumptions of normality and equal variances. The main advantage for nonparametric tests is that they provide more power than parametric tests when the samples are from highly skewed distributions, but they provide less power than parametric tests when the distributions are near normal. The *power* of a test is the probability of correctly rejecting the null hypothesis when it is in fact false. The computational formulas for the Mann-Whitney U test and t test for unrelated samples are found in most basic statistics books. The statistical procedures are also included in most statistical software applications.

Technology Note

Microsoft Excel provides statistical analysis tools in its Analysis ToolPack—including analysis of variance, the F test for homogeneity of variances, t-test, and z-test procedures. However, Excel's application for statistical analysis is limited (cf.*http://www.practicalstats.com/Pages/excelstats.html*). Alternatives are statistical software packages such as Analyse-it (*http://www.analyse-it.com*)—a statistical add-in for Excel. Analyse-it replaces Excel algorithms and provides additional statistical resources. Statistical software applications that stand alone include SPSS v. 13.0 and Minitab Release 14. Both SPSS and Minitab include spreadsheets and a comprehensive array of statistical options.

Tests for Related Samples

The t test for related samples is used to answer the question: Is an observed difference between two conditions within the same subjects attributable to chance? If not, the alternative hypothesis is accepted. In the case of related (correlated) samples, data are naturally paired. The data are naturally paired when the same subjects are measured twice, such as in the case of (a) pretest-posttest designs, or (b) same-subjects designs with two conditions. To correctly use the t test for related samples, several assumptions are critical. First, subjects must be randomly sampled from the population. Second, the two sets of scores must be correlated (related). Third, the sampling distributions must be normally distributed. The t test for related samples is computed as the mean of the differences in scores between pairs of subjects divided by the standard error of the difference (S.E.D.).

A case example is Hubbard's (1998) study of the effect of syllabic stress on stuttering behaviors. Hubbard recruited 10 adult stutterers as participants and asked them to read aloud 40 sentences that varied in locations of syllabic stress. Hubbard (1998) compared the frequency of stuttering with the same subjects in two conditions—stressed and unstressed syllables. The statistical analysis was accomplished by using a t test for related samples. Hubbard (1998) reported no significant difference between the two conditions ($t = -0.44$, $p = .67$). Hubbard's (1998) t test included both tails of the t distribution (two-tailed test), but Smith-Olinde, Besing, and Koehnke (2004) chose a one-tailed t test because they hypothesized "poor performance by the group with hearing loss [vs. the normal hearing group]" (p. 86). The Smith-Olinde et al. (2004) directional hypothesis increased the power of their statistical analysis in that the probability of rejecting the null hypothesis increased. If Hubbard's (1998) hypothesis was directional, how would a one-tailed test change the result?

The nonparametric alternative to the t test for related samples is the *Wilcoxon test for paired data*. The Wilcoxon test is an appropriate choice when sample distributions are highly skewed. The computational formulas for the Wilcoxon test and the t test for related samples are found in most basic statistics books. The statistical procedures are also included in most statistical software applications.

Tests for Differences Between Multiple Groups or Conditions

Most research in communication disorders has progressed beyond the stage where only two groups (experimental and control) or two conditions are compared to each other. Contemporary experiments in communication disorders are typically more complex because researchers attempt to account for the complexities of natural events. By far, the majority of statistical procedures reported in the Results *section* of articles in communication disorders are some variant of the analysis of variance (ANOVA) approach to statistical analysis (Meline & Wang, 2004). The outcome of analysis of variance is an F ratio, or F statistic. The F statistic is named in recognition of R. A. Fisher's contributions to statistics. The analysis of variance is so named because it compares variances in order to test for differences between means.

Analysis of variance procedures are accompanied by assumptions, similar to the assumptions for t-test procedures. The results of analysis of variance are less precise when

Technology Note

The Internet provides access to several online calculators for t-tests and the simple analysis of variance. The *Simple Interactive Statistical Analysis (SISA)* web page includes an interface for calculating t-tests with the input of means, sample sizes, and standard deviations. It also calculates confidence intervals. The SISA's web page is: *http://home.clara.net/sisa/t-test.htm*. Another online t-test calculator is available at: *http://www.graphpad.com/quickcalcs/test1.cfm*. It allows various data entry choices and the choice of related, unrelated, and Welch-Satterthwaite versions of the t-test. An online, interactive calculator for simple analysis of variance is available at: *http://www.physics.csbsju.edu/stats/anova.html*.

assumptions are violated. The general assumptions for analysis of variance procedures are as follows:

1. Data are continuously measured—usually an interval level of measurement.
2. Subjects should be randomly sampled from the population.
3. Data are sampled from populations with normal distributions, as estimated by sample variances. However, parametric tests are robust to violations of normality when sample size is large ($n \geq 30$).
4. Data are sampled from populations with equal variances, as estimated by sample variances. Parametric tests are especially vulnerable to violations of equal variances when sample sizes are unequal. *Levene's test* for homogeneity of variance is used to test the null hypothesis that multiple samples are equal.

Whereas the t-test procedure is limited to analyzing two groups or comparisons at one time, analysis of variance procedures permit the analysis of many groups or comparisons at one time. In the special case of two sample means, the analysis of variance procedure is equivalent to the t test, in other words, $F = t^2$. As is the case with the t test, there are many different analysis of variance procedures to match the many possible experimental designs in communication disorders. Analysis of variance procedures are classified as *one-way* (one grouping factor), *two-way* (two grouping factors), *three-way* (three grouping factors), and so on. Analysis of variance procedures with multiple factors are generally known as *multifactor analyses of variance*. Thus, analysis of variance is broadly classified as either (a) simple analysis of variance procedures, or (b) complex analysis of variance procedures.

Simple Analysis of Variance Procedures

The purpose of simple analysis of variance is to determine the probability that the means of some groups of scores deviate from one another by sampling error alone. To accomplish this purpose, analysis of variance separates variance into: (a) *within-group variability,* and (b) *between-groups variability*. Variances are partitioned so that researchers can ascertain how much of the total variance is attributable to sampling error and how much is attributable to the treatment effect. The *within-group variability* is the portion of total variance that cannot be explained by the research design. In the analysis of variance procedure, it is known as the *mean square for error* (MS_{ERROR}) and is the denominator in the F ratio. The between-groups variability is the portion of total variance that is attributable to group membership. In the analysis of variance procedure, it is known as the *mean square for effect* (MS_{EFFECT}) and is the numerator in the F ratio. Thus, the F statistic is computed as the ratio between MS_{EFFECT} and MS_{ERROR} as shown below.

$$F \text{ statistic} = \frac{MS_{effect}}{MS_{error}}$$

The two estimates of variance (MS_{EFFECT} and MS_{ERROR}) are compared in order to test whether the ratio of the two variances is significantly greater than 1. A case example is Erler and Garstecki's (2002) investigation of women's perceptions of hearing loss and hearing-aid use. Their purpose was to "examine the degree of stigma associated with hearing loss and hearing aid use among women in three age groups (35–45 years, 55–65 years, and 75–85 years)" (Erler & Garstecki, 2002, p. 83). As a preliminary to examining perceptions of stigma associated with hearing loss and hearing-aid use, Erler and Garstecki (2002) gathered demographic data from 191 participants. The demographic data for years of education, general health, and health handicap were measured on a continuous scale, so the researchers employed several one-way analyses of variance procedures to test for differences between the three age groups. Erler and Garstecki (2002) reported significant differences for years of education (F = 6.2, p < .01) and health handicap (F = 3.2, p < .05) but no significant difference between age groups for reports of health status (F = 0.053, p > .05). Based on the analysis of variance results, the researchers concluded that the women in the 75–85-year-old group reported less years of education and were more likely to report a health handicap. Did the researchers meet the assumption of normality? What information is needed to evaluate the remaining assumptions for analysis of variance?

A second case example is Stuart's (2004) investigation of word list equivalency for auditory testing in different noise conditions (signal/noise ratios). Stuart (2004) selected one-way analysis of variance procedures to evaluate the differences between noise conditions. However, the dependent variable was measured as "percentage of words correctly recognized,"—and data expressed as proportions typically require some transformation before the statistical analysis to satisfy the assumptions of analysis of variance. This is especially true when a large number of the proportions are small (< 0.20) or large (> 0.80). Stuart (2004) chose the conventional transformation for proportional data—the *arcsine transformation*. Arcsine is the trigonometric function known as the inverse sine. Following the transformation, Stuart (2004) successfully analyzed the data.

The nonparametric alternative to the one-way analysis of variance is the *Kruskal-Wallis Test*. It is used to compare three or more independent groups of sampled data—as in the case of one-way analysis of variance. The test statistic for the Kruskal-Wallis Test is H. The Kruskal-Wallis Test is typically used when samples are very small (n < 10) or when sample sizes are seriously unbalanced. The computational formulas for the Kruskal-Wallis Test and the one-way analysis of variance are found in most basic statistics books. The statistical procedures are also included in most statistical software applications.

Complex analysis of variance procedures. One-way analysis of variance includes one independent variable with several levels—but complex analysis of variance procedures include two or more independent variables (factors). By including two or more factors, researchers are able to evaluate the interactions between factors (*interaction effects*) as well as the separate effects of each factor (*main effects*). The presence of a significant interaction effect means that the main effects cannot be relied upon to tell the whole story. A general way to express interactions is to say an effect is modified by another effect. The term "interaction" was first used by Fisher, circa 1926.

Research questions in communication disorders may include more than one factor. A case example is an experiment reported by Turkstra, Ciccia, and Seaton (2003). They recruited 50 participants (13–20 years of age) including 24 females, 26 males, 21 African Americans, and 29 Caucasians. Turkstra et al. (2003) asked if race and sex groupings were related to frequency of conversational turns. To answer this question, the research team employed a multifactor analysis of variance procedure. Turkstra et al. (2003) reported a significant main effect for sex on frequency of turns (F = 5.66, p < .05). Males took significantly more turns than females. No other main effect was significant, and there was no significant interaction effect. What if the interaction effect had been significant? How would the researchers have interpreted an interaction between sex and race factors?

Turkstra et al. (2003) relied upon the main effect alone for their interpretation of results because there was no interaction effect, but factors sometimes interact to produce an effect. As an illustration, Table 9.1 depicts an interaction effect in a fictional study of aphasia treatments and time post onset for the initiation of treatment. In this case, subjects were given either treatment A or treatment B, and treatments were initiated at two different times—1 month post onset and 4 months post onset. As a result, the treatment effect was modified by the time post-onset for initiation of therapy. When treatments were initiated at 4 months, there was little difference between treatments A and B (82 vs. 80%). However, when treatments were initiated at 1-month post-onset, there was a significant difference between treatments A and B (80 vs. 92 percent).

To further evaluate research results for interaction effects, simple line graphs are useful for depicting the course of the dependent variable across two factors. The presence of interaction is indicated by non-parallel lines. If the lines cross, or if the lines would cross if extended, there is probably an interaction effect. The data reported in Table 9.1 are displayed as a graph in Figure 9.1.

The lines drawn in Figure 9.1 are clearly not parallel. This result is a strong indication that there is a significant interaction effect. Based on the fictitious data in Table 9.1, which treatment is most efficacious? Based on the same fictitious data, is it better to initiate treatment at 1 month or at 4 months post-onset?

When multifactor analysis of variance procedures identify significant effects, the location of the effect is not always evident because of the number of means being compared.

Table 9.1   An interaction effect in a fictitious study of aphasia treatments and time post-onset.

Time Post-Onset	Treatment A Mean	Treatment B Mean	Row Mean
1 Month	80%	92%	86%
4 Months	82%	80%	81%
Column Mean	81%	86%	

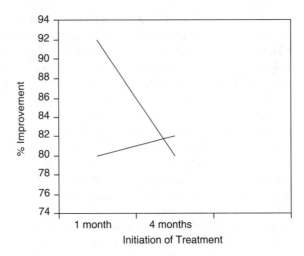

Figure 9.1   Visual representation of an interaction effect.

A significant main effect indicates the presence of at least one significant difference between means, but it does not identify specific pairs of means. The significant difference may be between one pair of means or several pairs of means. To remedy this problem, researchers utilize post hoc comparison tests which analyze pairs of means for significance. As a result, the post hoc tests identify the specific pairs of means that are significantly different.

There are a variety of post hoc comparison tests for analysis of variance. The most popular post hoc procedures are the *Bonferroni, Tukey, Newman-Keuls,* and *Sheffé tests.* A case example of post hoc comparisons is Stuart's (2004) experiment. In one aspect of the study, Stuart (2004) examined the effect of broadband noise with a signal/noise ratio of −5 dB on different lists of words used in auditory testing. The one-way ANOVA procedure was the choice for statistical analysis. The independent variable included four different word lists, so there were a total of six comparisons between means. Stuart (2004) chose the Tukey HSD (honestly significant difference) test for post hoc comparisons. As a result, Stuart identified three mean comparisons that were statistically significant. The remaining three mean comparisons were not significant.

The choice of one post hoc comparison test over another is not straightforward and is sometimes controversial. There is little difference between Tukey and Newman-Keuls post hoc comparison tests, but Bonferroni and Scheffé tests are criticized as being overly conservative. There are numerous Internet sites with information about post hoc comparisons and resources for their calculation. One is the *GraphPad.com* website. GraphPad.com includes an online post-test calculator (*QuickCalcs*) that accepts entry of mean square, degrees of freedom, and means for each paired comparison and provides online results.

The nonparametric alternative to the two-way analysis of variance is known as *Friedman's test.* Friedman's test is based on an analysis of variance using the ranks of the data, but it does not evaluate interaction effects. As is the case for other nonparametric tests, Friedman's test may be employed when assumptions about normality and homogeneity of variance are seriously violated. The computational formulas for Friedman's test and multifactor analysis of variance procedures are found in most basic statistics books. The statistical procedures are also included in most statistical software applications.

Tests for Analyzing Categorical (Nominal) Data

In some cases, researchers in communication disorders collect *categorical data* in the course of their studies. Categorical data are also known as *count data*—and the measurement is nominal level. For example, Erler and Garstecki (2002) collected categorical data from participants in their study of women's perceptions of hearing loss and use of hearing aids. The researchers asked participants to answer questions such as: (a) Are you currently married? (b) Are you currently providing care to others? (c) Are you currently employed? The *yes/no* responses classified participants by categories, such as *married, not married, employed,* or *not employed.* Thus, the data that were subsequently analyzed were nominal-level data.

The analysis of categorical data is accomplished with statistical procedures known as chi-square tests. There are a variety of chi-square procedures that are appropriate for different experimental designs, including between-subjects or within-subjects designs and unrelated-samples or related-samples designs. The purpose of chi-square tests is to determine whether the observed frequencies (counts) differ significantly from the frequencies expected by chance. Chi-square tests are accompanied by several assumptions and limitations:

1. Individual observations must be independent of one another, i.e., the response of one subject should have no influence on the response of another subject.
2. The observations for analysis must be count data, not percentages or other forms of data.
3. The sum of the expected frequencies must equal the sum of the observed frequencies.
4. The categories must be exclusive of one another.
5. The expected values for any one cell in the contingency table must not be too small (such as < 5), but the restriction varies with the type of chi-square test and the accompanying degrees of freedom.

Contingency tables are the rows by columns tables that are used to organize the data for chi-square analysis. An example is displayed in Table 9.2.

The general formula for the chi-square test is shown in the formula below, and the formula for calculating expected frequencies is stated in bold.

$$\chi^2 = \sum \frac{(O - E)^2}{E}$$

O = observed frequency; E = expected frequency

$$df = (columns - 1)(rows - 1)$$

Expected frequency for a cell = (column total × row total)/grand total

The data included in Table 9.2 were extracted from tabled values presented in the Erler and Garstecki (2002) article. Erler and Garstecki (2002) recruited 191 women with

Table 9.2   Contingency table (rows by columns).

	Young Women	Middle-Aged Women	Older Women	Totals
Married	40[A] (33)	42 (36)	21 (33)	103
Not Married	22 (29)	25 (31)	41 (29)	88
Totals	62	67	62	191

Adapted from Table 2, Erler and Garstecki, 2002, p. 85.
[A]Observed and (expected values)

age-normal hearing who were subsequently divided into three age groups: (a) younger women, (b) middle-aged women, and (c) older women. As a part of their investigation, the researchers analyzed demographic data that were gathered by a questionnaire. Only the data for one category (*married/not married*) are included in Table 9.2. The calculation of chi-square requires several steps.

The *first* step for calculating the chi-square statistic is based on the formula in bold—the column total (62) is multiplied by the row total (103) and divided by the grand total (191) to equal the expected value for *cell one* (33). The expected values for the remaining cells are calculated in the same fashion. The *second step* involves calculating the difference between the observed and expected value in each cell, squaring the difference, and dividing by the expected value. Thus, in the case of the first cell (*Young Women, Married*) displayed in Table 9.2, the computation is: $(40 - 33)^2/33 = 1.48$. The computations are performed for the remaining cells in like fashion. The *third step* involves summing the results from each cell of the contingency table. The outcome is known as the *observed value* of the chi-square statistic. The observed value is compared to the *critical value* for chi-square based on the appropriate degrees of freedom which are df = 2 in the example. The *critical values* of χ^2 are found in the appendixes of most basic statistics books.

Erler and Garstecki (2002) reported the result of their chi-square analysis as $\chi^2 = 14.9$, $p < .01$ (df = 2). Based on this result, the researchers concluded that there was a significant difference between age groups for the married/not married variable. Considering the Erler and Garstecki (2002) results, what age groups contained the greatest differences? Did the chi-square analysis satisfy each of the five assumptions for chi-square tests?

The chi-square test is an appropriate choice when sampling data are categorical such as in the case of count data. The computational formulas for a variety of chi-square tests are found in most basic statistics books. The statistical procedures for chi-square are also included in most statistical software applications.

CASE STUDIES

Case 9.1   A Quandary for Klein and Brown

Professor Klein and audiologist Brown recruited 20 older men and women to participate in an investigation of the effect of hearing-aid adjustment instruction on user satisfaction. The dependent variable is measured on a continuous scale. Klein and Brown's research question is: Will men and women differ in their user satisfaction? The researchers are uncertain about the choice of an analysis procedure—parametric or nonparametric. As the research consultant, what questions will you ask Klein and Brown to help them choose the proper analysis procedure?

Case 9.2   Inequality Dilemma for the Chavez School Research Team

The Chavez School research team randomly selected 100 kindergarten children in their school district as participants in a study of bilingual education. They divided participants into two groups—those assigned to bilingual education classes, and a control group in regular education classes. After collecting their data, the research team is uncertain about how to proceed because the standard deviations for the two groups are unequal ($SD_1 = 63.4$; $SD_2 = 72.1$). What is your advice for the Chavez School research team?

Case 9.3   Student Researchers Maria and Stephen Seek Advice

Student researchers Maria and Stephen devised a research design for a graduate course project that utilizes a survey questionnaire for gathering data. The questions in their survey instrument require yes/no answers. The independent variable is *class standing*—freshman, sophomore, junior, senior, or graduate. The researchers are uncertain about the quantitative analysis of their data. As a fellow student and ace researcher, what is your best advice? What are Maria and Stephen's options?

Student Exercises

1. Locate a research article in a recent journal and identify the quantitative analysis procedures utilized in the study. What were the levels of measurement for dependent variables? What quantitative methods were used? What was the sample size? Did the researchers satisfy the assumptions for their quantitative analyses?
2. Identify a recent research report with analysis of variance utilized as a quantitative method. Was the ANOVA procedure one-way or multifactor? What were the independent variables? Was there an interaction effect? What post hoc tests were used?
3. Locate a research article that includes a t-test analysis of two means. What are the values for the means and standard deviations of the two groups (or conditions)? Is the assumption of homogeneity of variance satisfied? If not, what alternatives would you have suggested to the researchers?
4. Identify a research article that includes a survey instrument in its *Methods* section. What were the dependent variables? What type of quantitative analysis (if any) was employed by the researchers? Did the researchers choose the proper analysis procedures? If you replicate their study, how would you improve the quantitative analysis of the data?
5. Locate a research article that includes a nonparametric procedure such as Kruskal-Wallis or Friedman tests. Why did the researchers choose a nonparametric test? Did the researchers make the proper choice?

10 Synthesizing Research in Communication Disorders

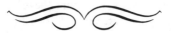

synthesis   (sĭn′thĭ-sĭs) *n.* to combine separate ideas or elements to form a coherent whole.

As a whole, research in communication disorders—and other disciplines—is poorly coordinated and sometimes disorganized. One problem is that many researchers work in relative isolation from colleagues with similar research goals. Though coordinated efforts are evidenced in urban research centers and within networks of colleagues, much research is planned and implemented by individuals or small teams of researchers who are not cognizant of ongoing research in other locales. Some disciplines have adopted *registries* of prospective and ongoing research, so that research plans of others are openly available to all. Thus, researchers are better able to plan and coordinate their own research efforts knowing what other researchers are doing. Lyons (2004) commented on the sometimes confusing state of the research literature in the social sciences—comments equally applicable to the research literature in communication disorders:

> Over the last 15 to 20 years, there has been an increased criticism of social sciences research because of the confusing state of the research literature. While one reviewer could find a set of studies that supported his viewpoint, a second reviewer commonly found several which did not support said conclusions. A common conclusion in reviews was "conflicting results in the literature, more research is needed to resolve this issue" which typically resulted in more studies which did nothing to clarify the issue.

The problem is particularly acute for clinical-outcome research—what speech-language pathologists and audiologists depend on for evidence-based practice. To alleviate the problem, Robey and Schultz (1998) proposed a "universal model for researching clinical outcomes" that includes five phases. A *phased model* is one course for organizing research outcomes into a coherent product.

A Model for Clinical-Outcome Research

The model described by Robey and Schultz (1998) provides a conceptual framework for the progression of clinical-outcome research from the early stages—focusing on exploration—to later stages focusing on refinement. Stage I research begins after the clinician-researcher formulates an idea. Robey and Schultz (1998) explained as follows:

> As an example of applying the model, consider that the genesis for an innovation in the treatment of [clients] arises from a clinical researchers' inductive reasoning based on experience and deductive reasoning based on expertise applied to observations of one or more patients. Having elaborated the initial insight to produce a basic treatment protocol, the clinician engages the model to pursue clinical-outcome research. (p. 795)

Phase I Clinical-Outcome Research

The goal for Phase I research is explorative—based on a tentative treatment protocol. Phase I observations are designed to detect the presence (or absence) of a treatment effect, as well as any negative consequences. The participants may not exactly represent the target population, and external controls may be lacking. Thus, Phase I studies are not rigorous experiments but are necessary to establish the ground rules for later experimentation. Typically, Phase I research is accomplished with small-group experiments (sample size < 30), case studies, and single-case experiments—A-B and elaborations of the A-B design. If Phase I results show no promise of a treatment effect, researchers may discontinue this line of research. However, if Phase I results reveal the prospect of a treatment effect, researchers may develop a protocol for Phase II research based on their observations.

Phase II Clinical-Outcome Research

Both Phase I and II are exploratory and prerequisite steps to a test of the efficacy hypothesis. Phase II goals differ from Phase I in that they aim to: (a) finalize operational definitions, (b) define the exact population of interest, (c) refine methodology, and (d) explore the treatment effect, both degree and permanency. Phase II research is typically implemented with case studies, small-group designs, and elaborations of the single-case A-B design.

Phase III Clinical-Outcome Research

Based on the findings in Phase I and II studies, Phase III clinical-outcome research aims to test the critical hypothesis and answer the research question regarding treatment efficacy. Phase III research includes large, representative samples of subjects (sample size > 30) and includes external controls in the form of comparison groups, such as no-treatment controls. A typical Phase III design is a pretest-posttest design with the comparison group receiving a different treatment.

Phase IV Clinical-Outcome Research

Phase IV aims to bridge the divide between research and practice—the transition from demonstrating efficacy in the laboratory to showing effectiveness in clinical settings. It is particularly important for researchers to collaborate with clinical-researchers to implement Phase IV clinical-outcome research. The focus of research in Phase IV may shift to specific subpopulations or may extend the treatment protocol to different populations. For example, Phase IV research might be extended to include different ethnic groups or different clinical groups. Phase IV research typically involves large-group designs but may include rigorous single-case designs with replication—typically with three or more subjects.

Phase V Clinical-Outcome Research

The focus of Phase V clinical-outcome research shifts to other treatment effectiveness issues, such as cost-benefit, consumer satisfaction, and quality-of-life issues. Phase V studies typically involve large-group and single-case designs but usually do not include a comparison group. *Synthesis reviews*—narrative and quantitative types—are particularly valuable means for combining the results from numerous Phase IV or Phase V studies.

The Robey and Schultz (1998) model for clinical-outcome research provides a framework for organizing research into a more orderly process. It is one means for organizing research outcomes into a more coherent product. Another means for organizing research outcomes is known as *synthesis review*. The synthesis review method is performed by identifying studies that have a common hypothesis, combining their results, and formulating conclusions based on the sum of results. The synthesis of results in communication disorders is accomplished by one of two methods: (a) *narrative review*, or (b) *quantitative review*.

Synthesizing Outcomes
by Narrative Review

The traditional method for reviewing the literature and synthesizing results is known as the *narrative review*. Kavale (2001) defined the narrative review as "a verbal report analyzing individual studies to reach an overall conclusion" (p. 178). The narrative review approach for synthesizing research in communication disorders requires: (a) a thorough search of the pertinent literature, (b) a qualitative analysis of the results of past studies, and (c) a conclusion based on the synthesis of results. An example is Glennen's (2002) narrative review of language development and delay in adopted children. According to Glennen, the primary goal was to "provide speech-language pathologists with an overview of linguistic, developmental, and medical issues that can potentially affect speech and language development in internationally adopted children" (p. 338). Glennen reported that little objective information was available, so a narrative review may have been the only available choice.

Eisenberg, Fersko, and Lundgren (2001) adopted the narrative review method to examine the use of mean length of utterance (MLU) for identifying language impairment in preschool children. Based on a comprehensive review of the literature, Eisenberg et al. (2001) concluded that MLU is not the best measure of utterance length for identifying language impairment. Narrative reviews are a valuable resource for synthesizing the existing literature on a topic, but the narrative review method suffers from some serious limitations. First, narrative reviews are especially vulnerable to the effects of researcher bias. If researchers have predisposed notions regarding the topic of synthesis, personal opinions may influence the conclusions. Second, synthesis by narrative review is prone to different interpretations by different authors. Two researchers may review the same literature and reach different conclusions. When the existing literature is sufficient in quantity and type, quantitative review methods are superior to narrative reviews for synthesizing research results in communication disorders.

Synthesizing Outcomes by Quantitative Review

The earliest known quantitative research synthesis is attributed to Karl Pearson, circa 1904. Pearson was a founder of statistics as a field of endeavor and is sometimes known as the grandfather of rigorous statistical evaluation for human behavior. The methods for research synthesis have improved considerably since Pearson's early efforts.

One of the simplest methods for the quantitative synthesis of research is known as the *vote-counting method.* In the vote-counting method, the results of selected studies are placed into one of three categories: (a) positive findings, (b) negative findings, and (c) nonsignificant findings. The category with the largest proportion of findings is asserted to support or refute the research hypothesis. The vote-counting method is limited because it is not sensitive to sample-size effects, and it does not evaluate the size of an experimental effect in a meaningful way.

An alternative to the vote-counting method for quantitative synthesis is known as the *combined-probability method.* According to Rosenberg, Adams, and Gurevitch (2000), combined-probability methods are the precursors to modern meta-analysis. Combined-probability methods were more powerful than vote-counting methods because they incorporate exact probabilities in the synthesis, thus accounting for different sample sizes. However, combined-probability methods do not quantify the size of experimental effects, nor do they evaluate heterogeneity among the studies (Rosenberg et al., 2000). The limitations inherent in vote-counting and combined-probability methods are overcome in modern meta-analysis methods. *Modern meta-analysis* combines measures of effect size from individual studies, achieves an overall measure of effect, and tests the significance of the overall effect.

Modern Meta-Analysis

Egger, Smith, and Phillips (1997) defined modern meta-analysis as "a statistical procedure that interprets the results of several independent studies considered to be 'combinable'" (p. 1533). The National Library of Medicine defined meta-analysis as "a quantitative method of combining the results of independent studies (usually drawn from the published literature) and synthesizing summaries and conclusions which may be used to evaluate therapeutic effectiveness, plan new studies, etc. It is often an overview of clinical trials" (National Library of Medicine, 2004b). Robey and Dalebout (1998) explained the need for quantitative synthesis in communication disorders as follows:

> As is true of any research question, compelling evidence for scientific conclusions cannot be accomplished through a single experiment or quasi-experiment. Science requires converging evidence from all independent experiments as the basis for a compelling conclusion. (p. 1227)

Andrews, Guitar, and Howie (1980) reported an early application of meta-analysis in communication disorders. They included 42 studies in a meta-analysis aimed at studying the efficacy of stuttering treatment. In recent years, the numbers of meta-analytic studies in communication disorders have increased—for example, Casby's (2001) meta-analysis of the effect of otitis media on language development, and Boutsen, Cannito, Taylor, and Bender's (2002) meta-analysis focusing on Botox treatment in spasmodic dysphonia. Modern meta-analysis is a powerful method for examining relationships in communication disorders, especially in the area of clinical-outcomes research.

Typically, synthesis reviews accomplish the following goals: (a) provide comprehensive summaries of research on a specific topic, (b) provide strong evidence for clinical decision making, and (c) identify future research needs. Synthesis by meta-analysis is based on the assumption that each study provides an independent (and different) estimate of the effect in the population. Thus, accumulating results across studies is expected to provide a more accurate representation of the relationship (between independent and dependent variables) than results from individual studies provide. In the special case of clinical-outcome research, meta-analysis has an advantage over large controlled experiments—a synthesis of several small studies may provide equally valid conclusions in a shorter period of time at less cost. Implementing meta-analysis in communication disorders requires four basic steps:

Technology Note

MeSH (Medical Subject Headings) is the National Library of Medicine's controlled vocabulary thesaurus. The MeSH thesaurus is used by the National Library of Medicine to index articles from 4,600 journals for the MEDLINE/PubMED database. MeSH descriptors help define searches for specific literature in communication disorders. MeSH facilitates PubMed clinical queries. The National Center for Biotechnology Information (NCBI) website includes a link to clinical queries using research filters. PubMed clinical queries can be performed with either: (a) a research methodology filter or (b) a systematic review filter—*http://www.ncbi.nlm.nih.gov/entrez/query/static/clinical.html*. The MeSH fact sheet and a downloadable electronic copy are available at the National Library of Medicine website: *http://www.nlm.nih.gov/mesh/meshhome.html*. Online tutorials for searching with the MeSH database are available at the NCBI website.

1. Develop a research hypothesis and define the eligibility criteria for inclusion.
2. Develop a search strategy and identify the studies for inclusion in the meta-analysis.
3. Convert the study statistics to a common effect-size metric.
4. Compute a summary effect and interpret its meaning.

Step One: Develop a Research Hypothesis and Eligibility Criteria

Initially, researchers should identify the parameters for the meta-analysis including: (a) the population to be studied, (b) intervention to be examined, (c) outcomes of concern, and (d) design of studies to be reviewed—randomized controlled experiments or quasi-experiments. Once the parameters are defined, the research hypothesis and questions should be evident.

Boutsen et al. (2002) employed the meta-analysis method to study the effects of Botox on patients with spasmodic dysphonia. They stated the study's purpose as follows:

> The purpose of this report is to review the BT [Botulinum toxin type A] efficacy data in adductor SD [spasmodic dysphonia] to determine whether and to what extent the aforementioned issues [BT treatment in SD is safe and improves vocal quality] make it necessary to qualify the view that BT is effective. (Boutsen et al., p. 470)

Based on the Boutsen et al. (2002) statement of purpose, what parameters can be identified? What is the common hypothesis—the hypothesis shared by all the studies included in the meta-analysis?

The criteria for including and excluding participants in a meta-analysis are known as *eligibility criteria.* The eligibility criteria are determined in the initial planning stage. They include factors such as: (a) the study design—experimental or quasi-experimental, (b) chronological window—years of publication, (c) language—English alone or others, (d) similarity of treatment, (e) completeness of information—summary statistics or primary statistic, (f) quality of method, and (g) combinability of subjects, treatments, and outcomes. Boutsen et al. (2002) described their study's eligibility criteria as follows:

> From the available pool of studies published between 1988 and 1999, 20 investigations were identified in which pre- and posttreatment measurements of SD speech or voice production were reported in sufficient detail to be included in a meta-analysis. These studies met the following additional criteria: (a) at least 5 SD participants sampled pre- and posttreatment, (b) the data pertained to the initial BT injection of patients who had not been treated surgically, (c) posttreatment measurements were reported short term and/or long term. (p. 477)

What are the Boutsen et al. (2002) eligibility criteria? What studies did they exclude from the meta-analysis of Botox and SD?

When evaluating meta-analytic studies, key questions to ask are:

1. Is the specific purpose of the review stated?
2. Are the hypothesis and research questions clearly and explicitly stated?
3. Are the eligibility criteria clearly and explicitly stated?

If the answers to these questions are affirmative, researchers typically advance to the next step—*searching the literature.*

Step Two: Develop a Search Strategy and Select Studies for Inclusion

Following development of the research questions and eligibility criteria, researchers should develop a strategy to search the literature. The goal is to assemble a database from which studies can be included or excluded based on the eligibility criteria. The initial database is typically much larger than the database studied. For example, Casby (2001) described his search strategy as follows:

> The following electronic databases were used in a literature search of primary studies of OME [otitis media with effusion] and oral language development from the mid-1960s to the present—*ERIC, PsychINFO,* and *MEDLINE.* The keywords used in the search were *otitis media* and *language.* The noted electronic databases are considered diverse and comprehensive in their coverage of the topic of OME. A total of 61 articles were identified via *ERIC,* 66 via *PsychINFO,* and 162 through *MEDLINE.* In addition, manual searches of the citations of the primary sources and other compendiums on OME were conducted to identify and locate further potential pieces of research. All of these sets were then further culled for studies that met the project's selection criteria specified below. (p. 67)

How many studies were identified in Casby's (2001) initial search? Following the inclusion and exclusion of studies based on eligibility criteria, Casby assembled a database of 32 studies. What was Casby's (2001) search strategy? Was the search strategy sufficient to identify all relevant studies?

A critical assumption underpins synthesis by meta-analysis—that is, the entire body of literature on the topic has been identified including published and unpublished works. Thus, it is important that researchers utilize all possible resources to establish their database. If researchers do not manage an extensive search of the literature, the validity of results may be compromised. This issue concerns content validity—the most common problem with content validity in meta-analysis is known as *publication bias.*

Publication bias exists as a threat because authors may not submit articles for publication (self-censorship) or editors may reject articles that report negative findings. Thus, articles that are published are more likely to contain positive results—consequently biasing the published literature. For example, Meline (2003) identified 201 presentations of experiments in an American Speech-Language-Hearing Association Convention Program, but only 60 of the experiments were published in the subsequent five-year period. Apparently, a substantial quantity of research is not published or may be published in unknown places.

The best way to avoid publication bias is to perform a diligent and extensive search of the topical literature. However, several acceptable post hoc procedures for evaluating the presence (or absence) of publication effects are available. Procedures for evaluating publication bias typically fall into one of two categories: (a) statistical techniques such as *fail-safe N* (Orwin, 1983), and (b) graphic techniques, such as the *funnel plot* (Egger, Smith, Schneider, & Minder, 1997). Robey (1998) explained funnel plots and their interpretation as follows:

> Publication bias, or the file-drawer problem (i.e., negative findings tend not to be published because authors chose not to submit or editors chose not to publish), can likewise threaten the validity of a meta-analysis. A plot of sample size over effect size is one means for detecting the possibility of publication bias (e.g., Greenhouse & Iyengar, 1994). In the absence

of publication bias, the plot should have the appearance of a triangle sitting on its base or an inverted funnel. That is, sampling theory would predict that (a) effect sizes derived from small sample sizes should be relatively variable compared to the more homogenous effect sizes derived from larger sample sizes, and (b) all should center around the same mean. (p. 182)

The other category of procedures for evaluating publication bias is *statistical techniques*. The most common statistical technique is known as fail-safe *N*. Robey (1998) explained his application of the fail-safe *N* method as follows:

> Another method for examining the validity of a meta-analysis is to calculate the number of null (i.e., [effect size] = 0.0) findings that would be necessary, if they existed, to diminish the value of [the combined effect size] to a critically low value (Hunter & Schmidt, 1990). For the within effects, the critical value of [effect size] for treated individuals is the corresponding value of [effect size] for untreated persons. The mathematics of Hunter and Schmidt (1990, pp 512ff) indicate that a total of 9 null findings in studies (i.e., each reporting [effect size] = 0.0) of treated aphasic persons in the acute stage of recovery would be necessary to lower the treated value of [the combined effect size] = 1.15 [observed value of treated recoveries] to the untreated value of [effect size] = 0.63 [observed value of untreated recoveries]. That is an unlikely prospect. (p. 183)

To establish a database of studies, Robey (1998) conducted an extensive search that yielded 55 reports of clinical outcomes that met the eligibility criteria. What is the basis for Robey's (1998) conclusion that nine null findings are an unlikely prospect? Robey (1998) utilized graphic (funnel plot) and statistical techniques (fail-safe *N*) as post hoc procedures. Why did he incorporate both graphic and statistical procedures?

Search strategies usually begin with electronic databases such as *PsychINFO* and *MEDLINE* because they index a large number of journals, and they are easily accessed. However, a thorough search strategy should include as many electronic databases as possible as well as a manual search. Electronic resources such as *ERIC* and *Dissertation Abstracts International* are an integral part to search strategies because they include unpublished materials in their databases. In addition, a search strategy should include a manual search of journals, books, and monographs to locate articles that may not otherwise be identified, with special attention to reference lists. Developing search strategies is an iterative process, one that requires multiple revisions. Typically, several trials are necessary before an acceptable database is attained.

To insure reliability, researchers typically develop a standardized recording form for data collection. Studies are subsequently selected or rejected based on the eligibility criteria. If quality of the study is a factor for inclusion or exclusion, *blinding* is a necessary precaution to insure validity and avoid experimenter bias. Before studies are evaluated for quality, the authors' names, institutional affiliations, journal titles (journal prestige may influence decisions), and other identifying information may be redacted.

When evaluating meta-analytic studies, key questions to ask are:

1. Were extensive search methods employed to locate studies?
2. Was an extensive search performed with appropriate databases?
3. Were other potentially important sources of studies explored?
4. Were reliability and validity issues addressed appropriately?

Technology Note

Meta-analysis procedures require intensive computations and complex manipulations of the data. The data collected for meta-analysis are typically entered into a spreadsheet format to facilitate analysis. Numerous statistical software applications are available for performing meta-analysis. One of the most complete applications is *MetaWin 2.0* (Rosenberg, Adams, & Gurevitch, 2000). The MetaWin 2.0 package includes *MetaCalc*—a stand-alone program that performs statistical procedures used in meta-analysis, such as converting primary statistics to effect sizes—and MetaWin, which is a comprehensive program for summarizing the results of multiple studies, calculating fixed-effects and random-effects models, and computing effect sizes and confidence intervals. MetaWin includes tests for heterogeneity and tests to evaluate potential publication bias. The MetaWin website is: *http://www.metawinsoft.com.*

Step Three: Convert Study Statistics to a Common Effect–Size Metric

Once the database is set, the goal is to convert statistics from each study into a common metric. In this way, the outcomes from each study can be combined into an omnibus statistic. The common metric is typically an effect size. The calculation of effect sizes is dependent on the data that is available in the primary studies. There are three categories of primary data: (a) summary statistics—mean, standard deviation, and sample size, (b) count data—two-by-two contingency tables, and (c) F, t, and X^2 statistics.

If summary statistics—mean, standard deviation, and sample size—are available, several alternatives are available for converting the summary statistics into effect sizes. A common effect–size metric is Cohen's d. It is expressed mathematically as follows:

$$d_{Cohen} = \frac{mean^E - mean^C}{\sigma}$$

$$\text{where } \sigma = \sqrt{\frac{(N^E - 1)(s^E)^2 + (N^C - 1)(s^C)^2}{N^E + N^C}} \tag{10.1}$$

To compute Cohen's d, subtract the mean of the control group (C) from the mean of the experimental group (E) and divide by the pooled standard deviation (σ). The result is a standard effect size that is interpreted like other standardized scores: An effect size of 1.00 is one standard deviation above the mean, an effect size of 2.00 is two standard deviations above the mean, and so on.

An alternative to Cohen's d is an effect-size statistic known as the *response ratio*. The *response ratio* (R) is the ratio of the experimental group's outcome to the control group's outcome. The response ratio quantifies the proportionate change that results from an experimental manipulation (Hedges, Gurevitch, & Curtis, 1999). It is expressed mathematically as follows:

$$R = \ln \frac{mean^E}{mean^C} \qquad (10.2)$$

According to Rosenberg, Adams, and Gurevitch (2000) the natural log of the response ratio (ln R) has "preferable statistical properties." The response ratio is easily interpreted. A value of zero indicates no difference in effects between experimental and treatment groups. Negative values indicate that control group effects exceed treatment group effects, and positive values indicate that experimental group effects exceed control group effects. As an illustration, Robey (1998) reported that the average effect size for treated individuals with aphasia was 1.83 times greater than that for untreated individuals with aphasia.

How would you interpret Robey's (1998) result in the context of treatment and no-treatment conditions? Is it a negative or positive outcome? How does this result relate to clinical practice?

A second category of primary data found in studies of communication disorders is the count data in two-by-two contingency tables. In this case, there are two groups—experimental and control—and two outcomes—response and no response. Table 10.1 displays a two-by-two contingency table with fictitious data.

Several effect-size metrics are appropriate for contingency tables, but a simple one that is easily interpreted is *relative rate* (RR)—rate of the experimental group relative to the control group. Based on the data provided in Table 10.1:

$$RR = P_T / P_C = 0.8 / 0.2 = 4.00$$

The interpretation of relative rate is straightforward. No difference between experimental and control groups is represented by 1.00. Values greater than 1.00 indicate positive trials—treatment effects exceed control effects. Values less than 1.00 indicate negative trials—control effects exceed treatment effects. A rule-of-thumb for evaluating the importance of the relative-rate metric is: 1.0 trivial; 1.9 moderate; 3.0 large; and 5.7 very large.

A third category of primary data commonly found in studies of communication disorders is *primary statistics* including F, t, and X^2. If summary statistics are not available to calculate Cohen's d or an alternative effect-size metric, primary test statistics such as F may be converted to effect-size metrics in two steps: (a) convert the primary statistic to a correlation, and (b) convert the correlation to a z-score. The conversion of primary test statistics to correlations is accomplished as shown in Equation 10.3.

Table 10.1

	Treatment	Control	Total
Response	8[A]	2	10
No Response	2	8	10
Total	10	10	20

[A]Number of observations

$$F \text{ statistic:} \quad r(eta) = \sqrt{\frac{F}{F + df_{ERROR}}}$$

$$X^2 \text{ statistic:} \quad r(phi) = \sqrt{\frac{x^2}{N}} \qquad df = 1 \qquad (10.3)$$

$$X^2 \text{ statistic:} \quad r = \sqrt{\frac{x^2}{x^2 + N}} \qquad df > 1$$

$$t \text{ statistic:} \quad r = \sqrt{\frac{t^2}{t^2 + df}} \qquad df = N - 2$$

A rule-of-thumb for evaluating the importance of correlation coefficients is: < 0.1 trivial; 0.3–0.5 moderate; 0.5–0.7 large; and 0.7–0.9 very large. Fisher's z-*transform*—shown in Equation 10.4—may be employed to convert correlation coefficients to a standard effect-size metric.

$$z = \frac{1}{2}\ln\left\{\frac{1 + r}{1 - r}\right\} \qquad (10.4)$$

When evaluating meta-analytic studies, key questions to ask are:

1. Were study statistics converted to a common metric?
2. Was the method for converting study statistics clear and explicit?
3. Were appropriate procedures used for converting study statistics to effect-size metrics?

Once study statistics are converted to common effect-size metrics, they are combined to form a *cumulative effect size*. Calculating a cumulative effect size is the last of the four basic steps for implementing meta-analysis.

Step Four: Compute a Cumulative Effect and Interpret It

The final step for synthesis by meta-analysis involves computing a cumulative effect and interpreting its meaning. The most common statistic for measuring a cumulative effect is the average value or mean. However, meta-analysis data typically include a mix of studies that are diverse in their settings, subject characteristics, and sample sizes. In addition, the overall quality of individual studies affects the aggregate result.

In general, large samples ($n \geq 30$) have smaller variances, and smaller samples ($n < 30$) have larger variances, but the mean statistic does not account for the differences in variation. The average of the cumulative result should give more weight to larger studies and less weight to smaller studies. According to Robey and Dalebout (1998), each effect size is weighted by its sample size so that the effects from small samples do not unduly bias the calculated value of the average. Thus, the individual results from studies are computed as the product of each effect size and its corresponding weight, and the cumulative effect is calculated as the average of the weighted effect sizes. However, a credible interpretation of the weighted cumulative average is not possible without examining the *heterogeneity* of the database in some detail.

The results of individual studies may be mathematically incompatible with the results of other studies in the database (Greenhalgh, 1997b). This phenomenon is known as heterogeneity. Some heterogeneity between studies is unavoidable, given the diversity of studies typically included in synthesis studies, but a significant degree of heterogeneity between studies may seriously undermine the interpretation of the cumulative effect. There are several procedures for measuring the degree of heterogeneity present in a sample of studies. A simple method is to visually inspect the data. For example, Egger, Smith, and Phillips (1997) recommended a graphic display of individual study results that includes means, standard deviations, and confidence intervals. However, visual inspection of the individual study results is not a definitive test for heterogeneity. A definitive test for heterogeneity may be computed as the *Q-statistic* (Hedges & Olkin, 1985), although there are other procedures available for testing heterogeneity. A significant Q-statistic indicates that the variance among effect sizes is greater than expected by sampling error alone (sampling or measurement errors). In this case, variance is caused by sampling error and the presence of confounding variables such as experimental biases or other threats to internal validity. If the Q-statistic is not significant, researchers may assume that the sample of studies is homogeneous, and the variance is attributable mostly to sampling error. If there is a significant degree of heterogeneity, researchers may examine their database more closely for the possibility of one or more moderator variables.

A *moderator variable* is an independent variable, other than the treatment variable, that explains a significant amount of the variance between studies. Robey and Dalebout (1998) explained moderator variables as follows:

> Because one or more sources of variation (e.g., severity of disorder, duration of disorder, age) influence the outcomes of primary studies, the average effect for all studies contributing to a synthesis is often a moderately sized effect with a broad confidence interval. A stratified analysis, separate analyses for each level (or class or category) of a theory-driven explanatory variable, may result in understandably different average effect sizes. Such a categorical independent variable (or one that can be made categorical) is termed a moderator variable. (p. 1231)

The presence of one or more moderator variables can significantly enhance the interpretation of meta-analysis findings. For example, Robey (1998) synthesized aphasia treatment outcomes from various studies. The cumulative effect for all studies was a moderate effect with a wide confidence interval. A further examination of Robey's (1998) data disclosed the presence of a moderator variable—*time post-onset for treatment*. Based on evidence for a moderator variable, Robey (1998) concluded that patients who were treated early (1 month post-ictus) demonstrated larger gains than patients who were treated late (12 months post-ictus). An analysis of the data is important for identifying possible moderator variables, but the analysis is limited by the number of studies included in a meta-analysis (Robey & Dalebout, 1998). Thus, researchers cannot inspect the data for moderator variables when the number of studies is small.

Statistical Models

Researchers typically adopt one of two statistical models to represent the data, based on the results of heterogeneity tests. The two general models are known as: (a) the fixed-effects model, and (b) the random-effects model. The *fixed-effects model* assumes that the variability of results between studies is attributable to random variation alone—more typical for randomized controlled experiments. Alternatively, the random-effects model assumes that the variability of results between studies is attributable to random variation plus the effects of confounding variables, such as experimental biases and other threats to internal validity. The random-effects model more often fits the data accumulated from quasi-experimental studies. The fixed-effects model is the more powerful model but not appropriate if the data are heterogeneous. Researchers may assign one or the other model to their aggregate data based on the results of heterogeneity tests.

The interpretation of the cumulative effect of synthesis by meta-analysis depends on the validity of the database, the calculation of cumulative effects, the presence or absence of moderator variables, and other factors. When evaluating meta-analytic studies, key questions to ask are:

1. Was the method for accumulating results from individual studies clear and explicit?
2. Were the methods for combining study effects appropriate?
3. Were the data tested for heterogeneity and an appropriate statistic model utilized for the analysis?
4. Were the data inspected for possible moderator variables?
5. Were interpretations and conclusions consistent with the results?
6. Were results discussed in relation to evidence-based practice?
7. Were implications for future research discussed?

CASE STUDIES

Case 10.1   Database Dilemmas

A team of researchers that includes an academic researcher and clinical researchers identified an initial database of 60 studies based on multiple searches in *MEDLINE* and *PsychInfo* databases. They have consulted you to help determine if the database is adequate for analysis. What advice will you offer to the research team? Once they have exhausted the search for topical literature, how should they proceed? What is the next step?

Case 10.2   More or Less for Professor Moore and Associates

Professor Moore and associates accumulated a database for analysis, and they tested it for heterogeneity. The result was a significant test for heterogeneity. They have considered adopting a random-effects model and analyzing the data accordingly. Inasmuch as you are the expert in meta-analysis procedures, they consulted you for an alternative course of action. What is an alternative to accepting the random-effects model? Is a reexamination of the studies in their database possible? What can Professor Moore and associates do to improve the database?

Case 10.3   A Problem of Incompatibility

Professor Tolkien and SLP Mathers have undertaken a meta-analysis of clinical outcomes for phonologically impaired children. They successfully established a database of 40 studies, but they are not sure how to convert the individual study results to a common metric. Some of the study results are expressed as means, standard deviations, and sample sizes alone. Other study results are expressed as F- or t-statistics with no means or standard deviations available. As a research consultant, what course of action do you recommend to Tolkien and Mathers? Can they find a common metric for the studies in their database?

Student Exercises

1. Search the current journals in communication disorders for a report of qualitative synthesis. What is the researchers' rationale for selecting a qualitative research method? Could they have performed a quantitative analysis of the data?
2. The Q statistic is one procedure for determining the heterogeneity of a sample of studies. What other techniques are available for testing heterogeneity? What are their applications and limitations?
3. Search the current journals in communication disorders and identify a report of synthesis by meta-analysis. What was the researchers' search strategy? How did they evaluate their database for a possible publication bias effect?
4. Identify a meta-analysis study in the communication disorders literature. What are the authors' interpretation of the data and their conclusions? Evaluate their conclusions for consistency with results and completeness. Did the researchers recommend future courses for studying the problem?
5. Identify a meta-analysis study in the communication disorders literature and evaluate its methodology. How did the researchers aggregate the outcomes from individual studies? How would you improve their method of study?

PART IV

Applied Research
for Speech-Language Pathologists
and Audiologists

11 Evaluating Research for Practice in Communication Disorders

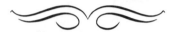

evaluate   (ĭ-văl′ yōō-āt′) v. to examine and judge carefully; appraise the value or worth of something.

The ability to access vast amounts of information in the 21st century is unparalleled in history, but not all information—whether research articles or other sources of information—is created equal, and not all information is good according to the National Information Center on Health Services Research and Health Care Technology (National Library of Medicine, 2004b). For these reasons, *information literacy* has emerged as an important goal for educators, students, researchers, and practitioners. The Association of College and Research Libraries (ACRL, 2000) issued information literacy competency standards for higher education that provide a framework for assessing information literacy in individuals. The ACRL published a definition of information literacy and emphasized the challenges that information literacy poses for society as follows:

> Information literacy is a set of abilities requiring individuals to "recognize when information is needed and have the ability to locate, evaluate, and use effectively the needed information." Information literacy also is increasingly important in the contemporary environment of rapid technological change and proliferating information resources. Because of the escalating complexity of this environment, individuals are faced with diverse, abundant information choices—in their academic studies, in the workplace, and in their personal lives. Information is available through libraries, community resources, special interest organizations, media, and the Internet—and increasingly, information comes to individuals in unfiltered formats, raising questions about its authenticity, validity, and reliability. In addition, information is available through multiple media, including graphical, aural, and textual, and these pose new challenges for individuals in evaluating and understanding it. The uncertain quality and expanding quantity of information pose large challenges for society. (Association of College & Research Libraries, 2000, pp. 2–3)

The Association of College and Research Libraries (2000) prescribed standards of information literacy for the following:

1. Determining the nature and extent of information needed.
2. Accessing needed information effectively and efficiently.
3. Evaluating information and its sources critically and incorporating selected information into one's personal knowledge base and value system.
4. Using the information effectively to accomplish a specific purpose.
5. Understanding the economic, legal, and social issues surrounding the use of information—accessing and using the information ethically and legally.

In regard to literacy and evidence-based practice, Nail-Chiwetalu and Bernstein Ratner (2003), remarked as follows:

[There are] direct parallels between evidence-based practice as endorsed by the [Certificates of Clinical Competence] and the information literacy competency standards. Importantly, it is difficult to achieve the goals of [evidence-based practice] if one cannot obtain and interpret the evidence appropriately. (pp. 166–167)

According to Law's (2000) scheme, *evidence-based practice* involves the systematic use of best evidence for solving clinical problems and includes eight steps to achieve an evidence-based practice. The eight steps are as follows:

1. Clearly identify the clinical problem.
2. Gather information from research studies about this problem.
3. Ensure that you have adequate knowledge to read and critically analyze the research studies.
4. Decide if a research article or review is relevant to the clinical problem.
5. Summarize the information so that it can be easily used in your practice.
6. Define the expected outcomes for the children [or adults] and their families.
7. Provide education and training to implement the suggested change in practice.
8. Evaluate the practice change and modify (if necessary). pp. 33–34)

To gather information about the problem, knowledge about available sources is necessary. There are two broad sources of information for evidence-based practice: (a) *raw evidence,* which is information that has not been subjected to expert review, and (b) *pre-filtered evidence,* which is information that has been reviewed by experts such as is the case for articles in peer-reviewed journals. However, regarding pre-filtered evidence, Beeman (2002) warned that research published in scientific journals gives the readers some confidence in the scientific credibility of research findings, but scientific credibility does not necessarily mean that the findings represent the truth. Both types of prospective evidence (*pre-filtered* and *raw*) require critical evaluation by consumers.

After identifying a clinical problem, students, researchers, and practitioners typically search databases for pertinent information. Modern technology provides computerized search engines that facilitate searching the databases with what are known as *key words*. Nail-Chiwetalu and Bernstein Ratner (2003) described their experience using different search engines to gather evidence about stuttering treatment as follows:

In our next search, we simulated the task of a student who wanted to know about treatment of stuttering using altered auditory feedback. Once again, we went first to Google. What we got here was a true mix, the kind that bedevils many professors attempting to mark papers. Of the 2,000 websites that were identified, a large proportion of the top listed sites on the first few pages were commercial ventures selling auditory aids for people who stutter. A few were sites featuring publicized aids on shows such as Oprah and Today. A few were unpublished conference papers. A few were chat rooms discussing personal experiences and devices. Taken together, they provided a relatively poor mix of resources for a student to determine whether or not auditory aids were appropriate treatment options for people who stutter. Next, we went to the database, Academic Search Premiere, and include[d] ERIC, MEDLINE, PsychInfo, and other major health-related databases in its search scope. We retrieved far fewer items, but the articles did tend to address whether or not auditory feedback affected stuttering frequency and severity. (pp. 176–177)

Locke, Silverman, and Spirduso (2004) adopted five basic questions as a guide for evaluating research reports, and their questions are a useful guide to evaluate research for practice in communication disorders. Greenhalgh (1997b) proposed an alternative set of questions that specifically target the evaluation of qualitative (as opposed to quantitative) research. Greenhalgh's (1997b) questions for evaluating qualitative research studies were as follows:

1. Did the paper describe an important problem addressed via clearly formulated questions?
2. Was a qualitative approach appropriate?
3. How were the setting and the subjects selected?
4. What was the researchers' perspective, and has this been taken into account?
5. What methods did the researcher use for collecting data—and are these described in enough detail?
6. What methods did the researcher use to analyze the data—and what quality control measures were implemented?
7. Are the results credible, and if so, are they clinically important?
8. What conclusions were drawn, and are they justified by the results?

The Locke, Silverman, and Spirduso (2004) taxonomy included five basic questions, applicable to quantitative and qualitative research studies. Locke et al.'s (2004) questions are: (a) What is the report about? (b) How does the study fit into what is already known? (c) How was the study done? (d) What was found? (e) What do the results mean?

What Is the Report About?

What is the report about? An answer is found in an article's *title, key words, abstract,* and *statement of purpose.* The *Publication Manual of the American Psychological Association* (APA, 2001) recommends: "A title should summarize the main idea of the paper simply and with style," and "A title should be fully explanatory when standing alone" (p. 10–11). For example, Ingham, Fox, Ingham, Xiong, Zamarripa, Hardies, and Lancaster's (2004) article was titled: "Brain Correlates of Stuttering and Syllable Production: Gender Comparison and Replication." What does this title tell you about the article, and what does it not tell you? The *key words* associated with Ingham et al.'s article (2004) were: *stuttering, brain imaging,* and *gender differences.*

Titles and key words are especially important because these terms are typically used to index articles in the repositories of major databases such as MEDLINE, ERIC, and

PsycINFO. Daniels, Corey, Hodskey, Legendre, Priestly, Rosenbeck, and Foundas (2004) chose the title "Mechanism of Sequential Swallowing During Straw Drinking in Healthy Young and Older Adults" for their research report. What does the title tell you about their study? Who were the participants? What were the experimental variables? What was the purpose of their study?

It is important that researchers state the *purpose* of their study in clear and concise words. A case example is Jupiter and Palagonia's (2001) article which investigated the use of the Hearing Handicap Inventory with elderly Chinese Americans. In this case, the authors addressed the purpose of their study in the first line of their abstract as follows: "The purpose of this study was to determine whether the Hearing Handicap Inventory for the Elderly (HHIE) screening version translated into Chinese can be used as a valid screening instrument for the identification of hearing impairment in Chinese-speaking elderly persons" (p. 99).

Was their purpose stated clearly and concisely? Do you understand the purpose of their study based on the statement in the abstract?

An article's *abstract* is a brief and comprehensive summary of the article. A good abstract is: (a) accurate, (b) self-contained, (c) concise and specific, (d) non-evaluative, and (e) coherent and readable (American Psychological Association, 2001). Ingham et al. (2004) wrote the following abstract for their article titled "Brain Correlates of Stuttering and Syllable Production: Gender Comparison and Replication."

This article reports a gender replication study of P. T. Fox et al. (2000) performance correlation analysis of neural systems that distinguish between normal and stuttered speech in adult males. Positron-emission tomographic (PET) images of cerebral blood flow (CBF) were correlated with speech behavior scores obtained during PET imaging for 10 dextral female stuttering speakers and 10 dextral, age- and sex-matched normally fluent controls. Gender comparisons were made between the total number of vowels per region significantly correlated with speech performance (as in P. T. Fox et al., 2000) plus total vowels per region that were significantly correlated with stutter rate and *not* with syllable rate. Stutter-rate regional correlates were generally right-sided in males, but bilateral in the females. For both sexes the positive regional correlates for stuttering were in right (R) anterior insula and the negative correlates were in R Brodmann area 21/22 and an area within left (L) inferior frontal gyrus. The female stuttering speakers displayed additional positive correlates in L anterior insula and in basal ganglia (L globus pallidus, R caudate), plus extensive right hemisphere negative correlates in the prefrontal area and the limbic and parietal lobes. The male stuttering speakers were distinguished by positive correlates in L medial occipital lobe and R medial cerebellum. Regions that positively correlated with syllable rate (essentially stutter-free speech) in stuttering speakers and controls were very similar for both sexes. The findings strengthen claims that chronic developmental stuttering is functionally related to abnormal speech-motor and auditory region interactions. The gender differences may be related to differences between the genders with respect to susceptibility (males predominate) and recovery from chronic stuttering (females show higher recovery rates during childhood). (p. 321)

What is your evaluation of Ingham et al.'s (2004) abstract based on the APA *Publication Manual's* criteria? Is the abstract accurate, self-contained, concise and specific, non-evaluative, coherent and readable? Rate the abstract for each of the five criteria along a continuum from poor (1) to good (5). Ingham et al.'s (2004) *statement of purpose* was given in the final paragraph of the article's introductory section as follows:

The present study replicates the Fox et al. (2000) procedure by comparing adult female stuttering speakers and normally fluent controls with previously studied male counterparts so as to (a) identify regions functionally related to stuttering across genders, and (b) determine the extent to which the regional effects associated with stuttering are gender-specific. (p. 323)

After examining an article's title, key words, and abstract, consumers should know if the article's content is relevant to their focus of interest.

How Does the Study Fit Into What is Already Known?

The answer to this question is found in the introductory pages of an article in what is known as the *Review of Literature*. The APA's *Publication Manual* (2001) recommends: (a) introducing the problem, (b) developing the background, and (c) stating the purpose and rationale in an article's introductory section. The literature review should describe past research results that are relevant to the problem at hand. The literature review is usually limited to current research but may include one or more classic studies if they are relevant. The literature review sometimes ends with a statement that addresses the relevancy of the current study. For example, Alt, Plante, and Creusere (2004) concluded their article's introductory section with a statement of how their study differed from previous studies and how their study was likely to contribute to the research literature:

Thus far, the literature has mostly provided information on how many words a child with [specific language impairment] can learn and how quickly he or she can learn them. Clearly, word knowledge is a process more involved than simply recognizing or producing a label. [. . .] This study addresses word learning in terms of (a) fast-mapping the phonetic strings that represent novel lexical labels, (b) fast-mapping semantic features associated with objects and actions represented by the novel lexical labels, and (c) the relative difficulty of mapping phonetic and semantic features for objects (nouns) and actions (verbs). (pp. 410–411)

When evaluating the introductory section of a research article, consumers should ask questions such as those proposed by Beeman (2002). For example, Beeman asked the following questions: "Does the study provide new knowledge? Does it test a new program? Does it contribute to what we know and don't know?" (p. 3). What are some other questions that you would ask in order to evaluate the content of an article's introductory section?

How Was the Study Done?

The answer to this question is found in the *Method* section of a research article. The APA's *Publication Manual* (American Psychological Association, 2001) explains the Methods section as follows:

> The Method section describes in detail how the study was conducted. Such a description enables the reader to evaluate the appropriateness of your methods and the reliability and the validity of your results. It also permits experienced investigators to replicate the study if they so desire. (p. 17)

The Method section typically contains three subsections with detailed descriptions of: (a) participants or subjects, (b) apparatus and materials, and (c) procedure—the step-by-step execution of the research plan.

Description of Participants or Subjects

A detailed description of subjects in research reports is critical for both the advancement of science and the advancement of practice in communication disorders. A detailed description of subjects permits a credible evaluation of results and allows practitioners to judge the transferability of results to their clinical settings. It also allows other researchers to replicate the study for confirmation of the results or to combine the results in the form of a *synthesis review*. A synthesis review is a study that aims to examine the results of similar studies to form a conclusion based on the collective results. A detailed description of subjects also permits other researchers to perform secondary data analysis. If the description of participants or subjects in a study is lacking, none of these goals can be successfully accomplished. Though each study is unique, the following questions represent the types of questions that consumers should ask:

1. What was the procedure for selecting subjects? Were subjects randomly selected? Did subjects volunteer to participate?
2. What was the procedure for assigning subjects to groups?
3. Is the control group equivalent to the treatment group?
4. Were subjects paid to participate in the study?
5. What are the demographic characteristics of participants—such as age, gender, and ethnicity?
6. Was there subject attrition during the course of the study?

7. What was the sample size? How many subjects completed the experiment? Is the sample size adequate for making meaningful conclusions?

The demographic characteristics of subjects are particularly important when they constitute experimental variables, such as *clinical status, disability, socioeconomic status,* or *sexual orientation*. When animals are experimental subjects, researchers should report characteristics such as genus, species, sex, age, weight, and physical condition. In all cases, researchers should provide enough detail for other researchers to successfully replicate the study and sufficient detail for generalizing results to clinical settings when the study has clinical relevance.

Daniels et al. (2004) described participants in their study of sequential swallowing during straw drinking as follows:

> Thirty-eight healthy adults were studied, including 20 right-handed young males between the ages of 25 and 35 years and 18 right-handed older males above the age of 60 years (range = 60–83). Fourteen young participants tested in a previous study (Daniels & Foundas, 2001) were included in the present study. Previous deglutition research has identified large effects (range – 0.90–2.0) when comparing the delay in onset of the pharyngeal swallow in older and young participants (Tracy et al., 1989). Power analysis revealed that an effect size greater than .89 would be detected with power equal to .80 with a sample size of 20 (α = .05), suggesting adequate power with the present sample. Exclusion criteria included a history of dysphagia, neurological disorders, chronic obstructive pulmonary disease, oropharyngeal structural damage, and a family history of dementia or Parkinson's disease. The study protocol was approved by the Institutional Review Boards at the Tulane University Health Sciences Center and the Veterans Affairs Medical Center in New Orleans. Informed consent was obtained from each participant. (p. 34)

What is your evaluation of Daniels et al.'s (2004) description of subjects? Are you satisfied with the demographic information that they provided? Why did they exclude participants with a history of dysphagia, dementia, or Parkinson's disease?

Daniels et al. (2004) provided a rationale for the number of subjects included in their study, but many researchers do not. Small numbers of subjects are especially problematic for group research designs because with very small samples, it is easy for coincidental relationships to emerge (Almer, 2000). Furthermore, Almer (2000) points out that a conclusion based on a very small sample with no basis in logic or theory is suspect. Very small samples are also problematic because real treatment effects may be obscured by the failure to reach statistically significant levels, such as the .05 confidence level. This scenario is possible because statistical significance depends on sample size. The smaller the sample size, the less the likelihood of identifying statistical significant effects.

Description of Apparatus and Material

The *apparatus and material* subsection in the Methods section provides a brief description of whatever apparatus and materials are used in the study. There is no need for detailed descriptions of standard equipment that is familiar to most readers. On the other hand, the apparatus and material should be described in detail if not commonly known. Though each study's apparatus and material are unique, the following questions represent the types of questions that readers should ask:

1. Are the stimuli that were presented to the subjects clearly described?
2. Can you clearly visualize the physical layout of the situation?
3. Is each instrument or material clearly described?
4. Is enough detail provided to determine if the instruments are reliable and valid?

Justice, Weber, Ezell, and Bakeman (2002) described the materials used in their study as follows:

> Materials included audiovisual equipment, one children's picture book, and a videotape for parent instruction. Reading sessions were recorded using two Panasonic VHS camcorders. To ensure that each dyad's book-reading behaviors were adequately captured during filming, one camcorder recorded a front view of the dyad and a second recorded a close-up of the open book. One children's picture book was used for all the reading sessions. *This Is the Bear* (Hayes, 1986) is a rhyming book that contains 24 pages, large narrative print, colorful illustrations, and numerous instances of contextualized print embedded within the pictures. The typical page contains between 8 and 10 words in the narrative and one or two instances of contextualized print in the illustration (e.g., in one illustration, a boy is waving down a truck by yelling "Stop! Stop!"). This combination of features was considered important for enhancing children's enjoyment of the activity and for providing ample opportunity for interactions regarding print. (pp. 32–33)

What is your evaluation of the Justice et al. (2002) description of materials? Why did they describe the children's picture book in detail? What apparatus or material in the study is assumed to be standard equipment—familiar to everyone—and what apparatus or material in the study is assumed to be unusual or unique to the study?

Description of the Procedure

The procedure subsection of the Method section describes what was done and how it was done. The procedure should be described in sufficient detail for replication by others and for transfer to clinical settings if the research has clinical application. The procedure subsection should: (a) summarize each step in the execution of the study, (b) describe instructions to the subjects, and (c) describe specific experimental manipulations. It should also include descriptions of control features that the researchers employed, such as randomization or counterbalancing techniques. There is no need to provide detailed descriptions of commercial tests or standard testing procedures that should be familiar to consumers. If a language other than English is used, the language should be specified. Though each study's procedures are unique, consumers typically ask questions as follow:

1. Are the instructions to subjects clearly described?
2. Is it clear how the dependent variable was measured?
3. Is the timeline for collecting data clearly described?
4. Are the manipulations of the independent variable(s) clearly described?
5. Are operational definitions for the experimental variables provided?
6. Are procedures free of the influence of extraneous variables?

Justice et al. (2002) described the *general procedures* in their study as follows:

Eligibility sessions took place in children's homes or on the university campus, based on parental preference. After eligibility was established, an individual data collection session was scheduled for each dyad on campus. This session consisted of the following. Parents first were asked to view the brief video training tape that demonstrated the use of print-referencing strategies. The children were engaged in an art activity in the same room while their parents were occupied. After viewing the video, print-referencing strategies were briefly reviewed by the examiner (the first author) using the picture book *This Is the Bear* (Hayes, 1986). To this end, each strategy was described again for the parents and two to three examples of each were demonstrated. Parents then were asked to use these print-referencing strategies while reading with their children. Parents were provided the book *This Is the Bear* and a set of written instructions that asked them to read with a normal volume and to keep the book flat on the table, both for video-recording purposes. This reading session was videotaped in its entirety and served as the basis for the analysis of shared book-reading interactions that occurred in this investigation. (p. 33)

What is your evaluation of the Justice et al. (2002) description of general procedures? Did they describe the procedure in enough detail to replicate the procedure in another research facility or within a clinical setting?

What Was Found?

The answer to this question is found in the *Results* section of a research report. The APA's *Publication Manual* (2001) describes the Results section as follows: "The results section summarizes the data collected and the statistical or data analytic treatment used. Report the data in sufficient detail to justify the conclusion" (p. 20). Researchers typically use tables, figures, photos, or other graphical means to enhance the readability and clarity of their presentation of results. The APA's *Publication Manual* also recommends *confidence intervals* as the best strategy for reporting statistical results. Confidence intervals are an alternative to traditional statistical significance tests of the null hypothesis (cf. Guyatt, Jaeschke, Heddle, Cook, Shannon, & Walter, 1995). Though each study's procedures are unique, consumers typically ask questions as follow:

1. Is there a clear presentation of the results in tabular or graphical form?
2. Is there a verbal description of results such as a statement of the difference between pre- and posttest treatments or a statement of the difference between experimental and control groups?
3. Are the correct statistical tests used? Do the researchers use distribution-free (nonparametric) tests when appropriate?
4. Are descriptive statistics appropriate for the dependent variable's level of measurement?
5. Are results reported in sufficient detail to answer each of the research questions?
6. Are the statistical analyses sufficient to address questions of *practical significance* and *clinical importance*?

The last question is an especially important one for consumers to ask because the answer is crucial for evidence-based practice.

Do the Results Address Practical Significance and Clinical Importance?

In order to evaluate research for practice in communication disorders, it is important to recognize the difference between the terms *efficacy* and *effectiveness*. Greenhalgh (1998) explained:

> There is a huge difference between efficacy (how well something works in the laboratory or controlled environment of the clinical research trial) and effectiveness (how well it works in the "real world" of the hospital ward, the clinic, the home and the community). (p. 3)

Though researchers may report significant statistical findings in their Results section, the results are not necessarily *clinically important*. Furthermore, the results may not be as effective in a clinical milieu—or may not be effective at all.

Bender, Cannita, Murray, and Woodson (2004) studied speech intelligibility in severe adductor spasmodic dysphonia (ADSD). Bender et al. (2004) described the study's purpose in the final paragraph of their introductory section as follows:

> Thus, the purpose of the current study was to investigate speech intelligibility in severe ADSD before and after Botox injection. We hypothesized that (a) intelligibility of speakers with ADSD before Botox injection would be significantly poorer than that of normal speakers, (b) following Botox injection, intelligibility of ADSD speech would significantly improve, and (c) intelligibility in ADSD would remain poorer than normal at 3–6 weeks following injection. (p. 23)

Bender et al. (2004) adopted a pretest-posttest design with Botox injection as the intervening treatment. As a control measure, the researchers included an age- and gender-matched comparison group. After describing their Method in detail, the researchers reported results with verbal descriptions and in tabular and graphical forms. Bender et al.'s (2004) primary result was their finding that the post-Botox condition was significantly greater (in speech intelligibility) than the pre-Botox condition ($p < .01$). The mean difference in speech intelligibility between pre- and posttest conditions was about ten percent (the percentages for speech intelligibility reported here are rounded to whole numbers). Based on this result alone, it seems that Botox may be an effective treatment for improving the speech intelligibility of ADSD speakers—or is it? Bender et al. (2004) did not report a confidence interval (CI) for the mean difference nor did they report an effect size. *Effect size* is a measure of practical significance (Meline & Paradiso, 2003), and confidence intervals measure the precision of a statistical estimate, such as the estimated mean difference between pre-Botox and post-Botox conditions reported by Bender et al. (2004).

If sufficient data are reported in the Results section of a research article, consumers can perform secondary statistical analyses. In the Bender et al. (2004) case, the researchers presented sufficient data to enable the construction of a confidence interval. The result is a 95 percent confidence interval (CI) = 4—17 percent.

How should the resulting confidence interval be interpreted? First, the most likely value for the difference between pre-Botox and post-Botox conditions is about 10 percent—the mean difference reported by Bender et al. (2004). However, the true difference may be as large as 17 percent or as small as 4 percent. Values further away from ten percent are increasingly improbable. A verbal description of results based on the confidence interval result is that ADSD patients who choose Botox treatment most likely (but not certainly) will experience improved speech intelligibility, but the size of the improvement in intelligibility may be small or large. The 95 percent confidence level means that there is a 95 percent probability that the true difference between means lies somewhere between the upper and lower boundaries of the confidence interval. In the Bender et al. (2004) case, the lower limit of the confidence interval is greater than zero, so their result is interpreted as a *positive trial*. If a confidence interval includes zero (i.e., the lower limit is zero or a negative value), the result is interpreted as a *negative trial*.

Another secondary statistical analysis that provides useful information for evaluating research for practice in communication disorders is known as *effect size*. Effect size (ES) measures are indicators of the *practical significance* associated with an experimental outcome. In the case of Bender et al. (2004), an effect size can be calculated as the difference between the means divided by the pooled variance. Bender et al. (2004) reported the pre-Botox mean (SD) as 79.43 (12.27), and the post-Botox mean (SD) as 89.86 (5.28). Given these values, the effect size (d) is calculated as follows:

$$d = M_1 - M_2 / \text{pooled variance} = -1.10$$

$$\text{where pooled variance} = \sqrt{[\sigma_1^2 + \sigma_1^2]} / 2 \tag{11.1}$$

In this case, the ES statistic is known as Cohen's d—a standardized effect size. The values of d are reported in standard units of measurement. Thus, a d value of 1.00 is equivalent to one standard deviation from the mean. The resulting effect size for the Bender et al. (2004) result is $d = -1.10$. The negative sign indicates the direction of the outcome—the difference between the mean percentages for speech intelligibility in the pre-Botox and post-Botox conditions. In this case, the magnitude of the experimental effect is slightly more than one standard deviation unit below the mean. An ES value of ± 1.10 is typically evaluated as a large effect—but it is better understood by considering the alternative interpretations displayed in Table 11.1.

Table 11.1 includes four columns of numbers with effect sizes from 0.0 to 2.0 in the leftmost column. The second column displays the percentile standings associated with the effect sizes in column one. Thus, an effect size of 1.0 is associated with the 84th percentile. The third column displays the percentages of overlap associated with the effect sizes in column one. For example, an effect size of 1.0 is associated with a 45 percent overlap (55 percent nonoverlap). *Degree of overlap* refers to the amount of variation shared by two variables, conditions, or treatments. Less overlap means a greater difference between treatments. Thus, effect size and degree of overlap are inversely related. The final column displays the probability of guessing group membership (such as experimental vs. control groups) from a single subject's score, rating, or performance—whatever value is assigned to the dependent variable. In the Bender et al. (2004) study, the effect size that described the magnitude of the experimental effect between pre-Botox and post-Botox conditions was 1.10. This ES value is equivalent to the 86th percentile and represents a 42 percent overlap—or a 58 percent nonoverlap. In terms of guessing whether a single subject belongs to the pre-Botox condition or to the post-Botox condition, the probability of guessing correctly is about 71 percent (7 out of 10 times).

Table 11.1   Interpreting Standardized Effect-Size Statistics: (a) Percentile Standing, (b) Percentage Overlap, and (c) Probability of Guessing Group Membership

Effect Size	(a) Percentage of Subjects in the Control Group below Average Subject in the Treated Group	(b) Degree of Overlap	(c) Probability of Guessing Group Membership from a Single Subject's Score
0.0	50%	100%	50%
0.2	58	85	54
0.4	66	73	58
0.6	73	62	62
0.8	79	53	66
1.0	84	45	69
1.2	88	38	73
1.4	92	32	76
1.6	95	27	79
1.8	96	23	82
2.0	98	19	84

Adapted from Table 1, Meline & Paradiso, 2003, p. 278.

What Do the Results Mean?

If researchers report results and analyses in sufficient detail, the conclusion to the research article is typically straightforward. However, if the results and analyses are not reported in sufficient detail, the research conclusions and associated clinical implications may be tenuous. The final section of the research report is known as the *Discussion* section. At this point in the presentation, researchers aim to examine, interpret, qualify, and draw inferences from their results. The conclusions should be logical, and they should be consistent with the reported results. The APA *Publication Manual* (2001) explained as follows:

> After presenting the results, you are in a position to evaluate and interpret their implications, especially with respect to your original hypothesis. [. . .] Open the Discussion section with a clear statement of the support or nonsupport for your original hypothesis (American Psychological Association, p. 26).

A factor that sometimes interferes with the formulation of meaningful conclusions is known as *confounding*. Confounding is a scientific term that refers to research studies in which there are two or more explanations for a given outcome (Almer, 2000). To illustrate, some patients complain of swallowing problems in the days and weeks immediately following onset of a stroke, but their dysphagic symptoms disappear after a short course of therapy. Based on these observations, should we conclude that the therapy

Technology Note

A recent survey found that effect-size (ES) statistics were included in less than half the articles published in ASHA journals, and only about half of those articles included interpretations of effect sizes (Meline & Wang, 2004). Thus, consumers may be left to evaluate the practical significance of research results on their own. In the case of treatment and comparison groups where means and standard deviations are reported, a standardized effect size can be estimated as the difference between the means divided by the standard deviation of the control group. In other cases, effect sizes may have to be computed from omnibus statistics—such as F or t statistics, which are frequently reported in the results sections of research studies. A downloadable (freeware) meta-analysis calculator that computes ES is available through page links at *http://www.lyonsmorris.com/*. An online effect-size calculator is accessible at *http://web.uccs.edu/becker/Psy590/escac3.htm/*.

alone is responsible for the improvement in swallow function or is there a plausible alternative explanation? Though each study's procedures are unique, consumers typically ask questions as follow:

1. Do the researchers discuss the importance of their *findings,* and are their claims consistent with the results?
2. Do the researchers discuss unexpected results and explain their meaning?
3. Do the researchers explain how their results fit with existing theories and how they are consistent (or inconsistent) with related studies?
4. Do the conclusions match the findings reported in the Results section?
5. Do the researchers discuss *cautions* or *limitations* in regard to findings?
6. Do the researchers discuss *clinical implications,* and are their conclusions valid?
7. Do the researchers recommend directions for further research?

In regard to the Bender et al. (2004) study, the researchers concluded as follows: "It is clear from these results that intelligibility is impaired in speakers with severe ADSD and that pharmacological therapy such as Botox injection provides a significant improvement in speech intelligibility" (p. 29). How would you evaluate this statement? Given the results, does Botox provide a significant improvement in speech intelligibility?

For consumers who are evaluating research outcomes for evidence-based practice, a critical question is: What is a clinically important change? Bender et al. (2004) reported a ten percent improvement in speech intelligibility following Botox treatment. However, the true improvement in speech intelligibility is probably somewhere between 4 and 17 percent, but what is a clinically important change? Is it 5, 10, 20 percent, or none of these values? A second question that is critical for consumers who are evaluating research for evidence-based practice concerns clinical economics. Is the benefit of the change cost effective, or is there an alternative treatment that may provide a similar benefit at a lower cost? In regard to the efficacy and cost of Botox treatment, Bender et al. (2004) commented as follows: "In the present push for treatment efficacy data, functional outcomes such as speech intelligibility can provide the justification for continued treatment via Botox, a very expensive form of treatment" (p. 29).

In this case, an important question is: How much change in speech intelligibility is needed to justify the high cost of the Botox treatment? When evaluating research for practice in communication disorders, it is especially important to ask the following questions: (a) Is the treatment transferable to my clinical setting? (b) How effective is the treatment likely to be in my clinical setting? (c) What are the economic considerations for my clinical setting?

Conclusion: Evaluating Research for Practice in Communication Disorders

The need for critical evaluation of research outcomes for practice in communication disorders is evident (cf. Reilly, Douglas, & Oates, 2004). To this end, there are many resources available to speech-language pathologists and audiologists that assist the process of transferring research results to practice. One such resource is in the form of a *checklist*. Inasmuch as *evidence grading* is an important aspect of evaluating research for practice, checklists are a means for grading the ability of research to predict the effectiveness of clinical practice.

Table 11.2 displays a checklist for evaluating the introduction, method, results, and discussion sections of research articles in communication disorders. Alternative checklists are available at the *Evidence Based Medicine Tool Kit* website: *http://www.med.ualberta.ca/ebm*. The EBM Toolkit includes worksheets for evaluating articles about therapy and/or diagnostic tests.

CASE STUDIES

Case 11.1   Professor Matlin's Dilemma

Professor Matlin and two clinical assistants completed an investigation to identify which of two treatments is the better one for improving speech fluency. Based on their pretest-posttest results, Treatment B had an 18 percent improvement overall, and Treatment A resulted in a 14 percent improvement. Which is the more efficacious treatment? What other considerations should be taken into account in their discussion of clinical implications?

Case 11.2   Collaborating for Reading Fluency

Dr. Gary and SLP Ruth are collaborating in a research project designed to identify the best protocol for improving third-grade children's reading fluency. Both of the treatments (*modeling* and *unison reading*) resulted in statistically significant improvements in reading fluency. As a research consultant, you are asked to help them with the interpretation of results. What is your advice for Dr. Gary and SLP Ruth?

Table 11.2   Checklist for Evaluating Research Articles for Practice in Communication Disorders.

Introduction Section: Review of the Literature and Purpose

1. Is the problem clearly identified at the beginning?	[ ]Yes	[ ]No	[ ]N/A
2. Is the review of literature selective, current and critical?	[ ]Yes	[ ]No	[ ]N/A
3. Does the literature review focus on research findings rather than opinion?	[ ]Yes	[ ]No	[ ]N/A
4. Does the purpose, research questions, and hypothesis flow logically from the introduction?	[ ]Yes	[ ]No	[ ]N/A
5. Are the research questions clearly written and operational?	[ ]Yes	[ ]No	[ ]N/A

Method Section: Materials, Procedures, and Participants

6. Are materials and any apparatus described in detail?	[ ]Yes	[ ]No	[ ]N/A
7. Are instruments properly calibrated and reliable?	[ ]Yes	[ ]No	[ ]N/A
8. Are human observers (judges) properly trained and reliable?	[ ]Yes	[ ]No	[ ]N/A
9. Are samples of questions, or directions provided?	[ ]Yes	[ ]No	[ ]N/A
10. Is there evidence of informed consent?	[ ]Yes	[ ]No	[ ]N/A
11. Are procedures described in detail?	[ ]Yes	[ ]No	[ ]N/A
12. Are treatments described in detail?	[ ]Yes	[ ]No	[ ]N/A
13. Were "blinding" procedures used?	[ ]Yes	[ ]No	[ ]N/A
14. Is the experimental setting described in detail?	[ ]Yes	[ ]No	[ ]N/A
15. Were subjects randomly assigned to groups or matched on critical variables?	[ ]Yes	[ ]No	[ ]N/A
16. Is the sampling procedure described in detail?	[ ]Yes	[ ]No	[ ]N/A
17. Were subjects randomly selected from the population?	[ ]Yes	[ ]No	[ ]N/A
18. Is the sample adequate for generalizing results to others?	[ ]Yes	[ ]No	[ ]N/A
19. Is the sample size adequate for the research purpose?	[ ]Yes	[ ]No	[ ]N/A
20. Are participants described in detail?	[ ]Yes	[ ]No	[ ]N/A

Results Section: Statistics, Interpretation, and Presentation

21. Are results clearly stated?	[ ]Yes	[ ]No	[ ]N/A
22. Are results adequately interpreted?	[ ]Yes	[ ]No	[ ]N/A
23. Are the statistical tests appropriate?	[ ]Yes	[ ]No	[ ]N/A
24. Are effect sizes included with interpretation?	[ ]Yes	[ ]No	[ ]N/A
25. Do the results directly relate to the research questions?	[ ]Yes	[ ]No	[ ]N/A

(con't.)

Table 11.2   *Continued*

Discussion/Conclusion Section: Limitations and Clinical Implications

26. Are the purpose and research questions restated?	[ ]Yes	[ ]No	[ ]N/A
27. Are limitations of the research design discussed?	[ ]Yes	[ ]No	[ ]N/A
28. Are results related to the review of literature?	[ ]Yes	[ ]No	[ ]N/A
29. Are clinical implications of results discussed?	[ ]Yes	[ ]No	[ ]N/A
30. Are future research needs discussed?	[ ]Yes	[ ]No	[ ]N/A

Case 11.3   Implications for Evidence-Based Practice?

As an expert reviewer for the journal *Language, Speech, and Hearing Services in Schools*, you are asked to critically review the manuscript for a research report. The manuscript's authors found a 10 percent difference between their pretest and posttest conditions and concluded that the treatment is an effective one that should be utilized by practitioners, but the justification for their conclusions is weak. What can you recommend to the authors to improve the reporting of results and improve their discussion of clinical implications?

Student Exercises

1. Develop a *checklist* for evaluating the content of a quantitative research report, a qualitative research report, or both.
2. Select a journal issue, such as the April issue of *Language, Speech, and Hearing Services in Schools,* and evaluate the titles for each article included in the issue. For titles that you evaluate as "poor," revise the titles so that they better satisfy the APA *Publication Manual's* criteria.
3. Select a journal issue, such as the fall issue of *Contemporary Issues in Communication Science and Disorders* (National Student Speech Language Hearing Association Journal), choose a research article, and evaluate its abstract. How would you rewrite the article's abstract to improve it?
4. Select a journal issue, such as the May issue of the *American Journal of Speech-Language Pathology,* choose an article, and evaluate its introductory section. Do the authors address the relevancy of their research? Does their literature review provide an adequate background for the focus of the study?
5. Select a journal issue, such as the August issue of the *Journal of Speech, Language, and Hearing Research,* and evaluate the researchers' conclusions. Did the researchers answer all of the research questions posed in the introductory section? Are the conclusions supported by the results of the study?

CHAPTER

12

Writing for Research in Communication Disorders

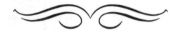

disseminate   (dĭ-sĕm′ə-nāt) *v.* to spread widely; to diffuse; to promulgate.

The research process involves planning, implementing, and dissemination. *Dissemination* is the act of sharing research methods, results, and conclusions with colleagues and others. Whereas the planning and implementation phases of research are relatively private enterprises, writing is a social enterprise and "a bold attempt to be part of our discourse community" (Academic Writing for Publication, 2002). The *discourse community* in communication disorders consists of academic teachers, scientists, practitioners, and students. These individuals comprise the audience for listening, reading, and evaluating research in communication disorders.

Researchers disseminate their research products for one or more reasons: (a) to contribute to the scientific foundation in communication disorders, (b) to stimulate further research in their area of study, and (c) to test their results and conclusions within the discourse community. The members of the discourse community—teachers, scientists, practitioners, and students—ultimately determine the worth of a research product. For example, researchers' success can be measured by *citation rate*—the number of times a research product is referenced by members of the discourse community. Another indicator of success is the use of the research product in speech-language pathology and audiology practices. However, some research results go unpublished or are otherwise not available for review by the discourse community. For example, mainstream journals typically publish less than half of the research presented at professional conventions (Meline, 2003). Thus, many research findings go unreported for one reason or another. The most likely reasons for not reporting research results are: (a) editorial rejections, (b) editorial censorship, or (c) self-censorship. According to McGue (2000), *editorial rejections* occur because of a lack of theoretical significance or some limitation in a research study's methodology. Controversial issues are the cause of rejection in the case of *editorial*

181

Technology Note

The thesis is a special case of writing in communication disorders. Waddell (2004) offered a metaphoric connection between thesis and Theseus—the mystical hero of ancient Greece who traversed the Cretan Labyrinth by following a thread. Like the labyrinth of old, the thesis is a labyrinth of ideas connected by a thread of thought that permits writers and readers to find the way. A thesis is a well-written analytical essay that addresses a research topic. A good thesis is: (a) clearly defined, (b) adequately focused, (c) well supported, and (d) high in the orders of knowledge (Waddell, 2004). Many resources are available via the internet to help thesis writers. For example, MIT's website advises thesis writers to think of the thesis as a series of small and related tasks: *http://web.mit.edu/Writing_Types/writingthesis.html*. Thesis writing resources are also available at internet sites such as the University of Kansas Writing Center: *http://www.writing.ku.edu/students/docs/thesis.html*; and the University of Wisconsin-Madison's Writing Center: *http://www.wisc.edu/writing/Handbook/Thesis.html*.

censorship. Self-censorship occurs when researchers choose not to report their publishable findings. The latter reason for not reporting research results (self-censorship) raises some ethical concerns as follows:

> For example, some individuals agree to participate in a research investigation only because they believe doing so contributes to a larger societal good. Failure to publish denies them the opportunity to fulfill that intention. Most significant, censoring certain research findings has the effect of producing biases and distortions in the research record. (McGue, 2000, p. 87)

Clearly, anyone engaged in the research enterprise has a duty to report research results in some form or fashion if possible.

Though researchers typically find the planning and execution phases of research to be exciting and challenging, the writing phase may seem tedious and dull. Sternberg (1993) observed this phenomenon with students who were completing research projects as follows:

> Many students lose interest in their research projects as soon as the time comes to write about them. Their interest is in planning for and making new discoveries, not in communicating their discoveries to others. A widely believed fallacy underlies their attitudes. The fallacy is that the discovery process ends when the communication process begins. Although the major purpose of writing a paper is to communicate your thoughts to others, another important purpose is to help you form and organize your thoughts. (p. 5)

Indeed, the process of writing is more than just a means to disseminate research products to the discourse community. Rather, writing is a recursive process that helps researchers generate new ideas and rethink old notions as they write.

The general goal for writing and presenting research in communication disorders is to publish or disseminate research products for review by the discourse community. However, writing has at least four specific goals as follow:

1. To inform—present the relevant facts.
2. To explain the relevant facts.
3. To interrelate the relevant facts—past and present.
4. To persuade the audience that the authors' explanation is the best explanation from among the plausible alternative explanations.

Each of these goals is equally important for successfully disseminating research products to the discourse community in communication disorders.

Writing is a creative process, but instruction and practice help to teach style and the mechanics of writing. The writing process as described by Emig (1971) and others is not a linear process beginning to end—but a recursive process with endless loops. The five stages of the writing process are: (a) prewriting, (b) writing/drafting, (c) rewriting/revision, (d) editing, and (e) publication/presentation.

The Prewriting/Planning Stage

Bem (2004) posed the rhetorical question: "For whom should you write?" According to Bem's (2004) philosophy, good writing is good teaching. Bem (2004) advised authors as follows:

> Direct your research writing to the student in Psychology 101, your colleague in the Art History Department, and your grandmother. No matter how technical or abstruse your article is in its particulars, intelligent non-[researchers] with no expertise in statistics or experimental design should be able to comprehend the broad outlines of what you did and why. (p. 189)

Clearly, the broad discourse community is the preferred target audience for writing level and style—not colleagues in the sciences. It also benefits evidence-based practice if researchers write papers to satisfy the needs of practitioners as well as academics (cf. Meline & Paradiso, 2003).

The *prewriting/planning stage* is a time to generate ideas and mentally rehearse the organization and writing of the research product. Sternberg (1993) posited what he considered *eight common misconceptions* about research papers as follows:

Misconception 1. Writing the [research] paper is the most routine, least creative aspect of the scientific enterprise, requiring much time but little imagination.

Misconception 2. The important thing is what you say, not how you say it.

Misconception 3. Longer papers are better papers, and more papers are better yet.

Misconception 4. The main purpose of a [research] paper is the presentation of facts, whether newly established (as in reports of experiments) or well established (as in literature reviews).

Misconception 5. The distinction between scientific writing, on the one hand, and advertising or propaganda, on the other hand, is that the purpose of scientific writing is to inform whereas the purpose of advertising or propaganda is to persuade.

Misconception 6. A good way to gain acceptance of your theory is by refuting someone else's theory.

Misconception 7. Negative results that fail to support the researcher's hypothesis are every bit as valuable as positive results that do not support the researcher's hypothesis.

Misconception 8. The logical development of ideas in a [research] paper reflects the historical development of ideas in the [researcher's] head. (Sternberg, 1993, pp. 5–13)

Technology Note

The internet offers a variety of online tutorials—instructional aids for writing and presenting research in communication disorders. A series of online tutorials at the KU Medical Center include modules for developing effective oral presentations, designing effective visual aids, and creating effective poster presentations: *http://www.kumc.edu/SAH/OTEd/jradel/effective.html*. The American Speech-Language-Hearing Association *Convention Presentation Site* (*http://www.asha.org/about/events/convention/papers*) includes "tip sheets" for all types of presentations. Online instructional aids are also available for developing writing skills such as the Purdue University *Online Writing Lab* (OWL): *http://owl.english.purdue.edu/* and the University of Missouri *Online Writery: http://www.missouri.edu/~writery*. *The Online Writery* provides an evaluation of writing samples with interactive feedback.

In what way is each of Sternberg's eight statements a misconception? After answering, compare your answers to Sternberg's (1993) comments regarding each of the eight misconceptions.

The journals published by the American Speech-Language-Hearing Association and most behavioral and social science periodicals expect contributors to adopt the style prescribed in the APA *Publication Manual* (American Psychological Association, 2001). According to the APA *Publication Manual's* guidelines, research papers should include: (a) an *Introduction*, (b) a *Method section*, (c) a *Results section*, (d) a *Discussion section*, (e) an *Abstract*, (f) a *Title*, and (g) a list of *References*. However, Sternberg (1993) points out that the steps followed in planning and carrying out research do not neatly correspond to the successive sections of the research paper. Rather, authors may write one or another section first (or last) depending on their personal style, though writing sections such as results clearly facilitates writing subsequent sections of the research paper such as the discussion. There is no preset length of time prescribed for prewriting and planning activities, but the better the plan, the easier the task of writing and drafting the research product. The *writing and drafting stage* follows the prewriting and planning activities in the first stage of writing research in communication disorders.

The Writing/Drafting Stage

Most important to achieving good scientific writing are accuracy and clarity according to Bem (2004). To write clearly, authors should first organize their research product and then adopt a simple and direct writing style (Bem, 2004). Sternberg (1992) offered 21 tips for better writing including 7 tips that specifically addressed the content of a research paper as follows:

1. Start strong.
2. Tell readers why they should be interested.

3. Make sure that the article does what it says it will do.
4. Make sure that the literature review is focused, reasonably complete, and balanced.
5. Always explain what your results mean—don't force the reader to decipher them.
6. Be sure to consider alternative interpretations of the data.
7. End strongly and state a clear take-home message. (pp. 12–13)

Authors should also be alert to the possibility of plagiarism. According to McGue (2000), plagiarism occurs when the words, ideas, or contributions of others (or self) are taken from speech or writing without proper citation or other acknowledgment. Authors are expected to properly cite their own work as well as others' works. Otherwise, authors are guilty of *self-plagiarism* and possibly copyright infringement. A *copyright release* is necessary to reproduce large amounts of material from published sources, such as tables, figures, or long quotes from books, monographs, and articles.

Writing the Introduction

According to the APA *Publication Manual* (American Psychological Association, 2001), the introduction of a research paper should: (a) introduce the problem, (b) develop the background, and (c) state the purpose and rationale. If the research method is qualitative, Pyrczak and Bruce (2003) suggested that authors consider discussing their choice of a qualitative design over a quantitative design in their Introduction.

To strengthen the opening, Bem (2004) suggested that authors open with a statement about people or animals, rather than open with statements about speech-language pathologists, audiologists, or their research. Furthermore, Sternberg (1992) recommended that authors open their research paper by telling readers what the article is about in a provocative way that catches their attention. Sternberg (1992) suggested a strong start that asks a question or states a problem pertinent to the theme of the article. Williams (2000) provided an example of a strong opening paragraph with a series of questions in her research paper, such as the following question: "Is one intervention approach suited for children of varying degrees of phonological impairment?" (p. 289). In similar fashion, Kamhi (2004) opened his article with a series of questions, such as the following: "Why do some terms, labels, ideas, and constructs prevail where others fail to gain acceptance? (p. 105).

Walters and Chapman (2000) illustrated a strong start of a different kind. They opened their research paper as follows:

Comprehension monitoring (Markman, 1977) is a necessary language skill in the classroom, as it is important for children to assess their own understanding of task instructions and teaching content (Paul, 1995). This metacognitive skill of monitoring comprehension is made up of two parts: Detecting a comprehension problem and indicating the problem to the speaker (Dollaghan, 1987). Dollaghan and Kaston (1986) propose[d] a comprehension monitoring intervention program for first-graders with specific language impairment that sequences the goals of monitoring acoustic distortions, inadequate content, and excessively lengthy and complex commands. This study examines whether Dollaghan and Kaston's (1986) sequence of goals corresponds to a developmental effect measures at ages three, six, and nine. (Walters & Chapman, p. 48)

Walters and Chapman's (2000) opening paragraph was strong in that it clearly informed readers about the research purpose. Asking questions, telling the reader what the paper is about, and stating the problem in the opening paragraph are writing techniques that help to get readers' attention. The Introduction of the research paper continues beyond the opening paragraph with a review of the pertinent literature (background) and a statement of the research purpose and rationale. Authors should demonstrate some logical connection between the previous literature and the present work. The *Introduction* typically ends with a statement of the hypothesis or a list of the questions that the researchers expect to answer.

Writing the Research Method

The Method includes a description of the participants, the apparatus and materials used, and the procedures followed to collect data. Sufficient detail in descriptions of participants/subjects is required to permit others to replicate the study. Thus, it is important to describe the subjects' ethnicity, gender, age, intelligence, socioeconomic status, and other characteristics—especially those that may interact with the experimental variables. Researchers should describe in detail the apparatus and materials used in the study, if atypical. If the apparatus and materials are common enough to be familiar to most readers, there is no need to describe them in detail. Finally, authors should describe the execution of the research step-by-step. It is necessary to describe the procedure in sufficient detail to permit others to replicate the method.

Jarvis, Merriman, Barnett, Hanba, and Van Haitsma (2004) reported three experiments in one paper, and they described the participants in one of their experiments as follows:

> Participants were 60 preschoolers and kindergartners ($M = 4;9$, range = $3;10 - 6;4$, all but 2 were 4 or 5 years old; PPVT-R $M = 94$, $SD = 14$) from predominately middle- to upper-middle-class families. Ten boys and 10 girls were assigned to each condition. (p. 400)

Did Jarvis and fellow researchers describe subjects in sufficient detail for a systematic replication of the experiment? What details, if any, are lacking in their description of subjects?

Writing the Research Results

The APA *Publication Manual* (American Psychological Association, 2001) specifies that the Results section should summarize the data collected and the statistics or data analysis used. In addition, authors should include tables and figures to display results. According to the APA *Publication Manual*, authors should also report statistical significance, confidence intervals, and effect size.

Researchers should not wait until the Discussion section to explain their results. Rather, they should interpret the results as they present them in the Results section of the research paper. Bem (2004) argued that descriptive results are more important than statistical results. He also recommended that researchers first state a result and then give its statistical significance—and in no case should the statistical test stand alone without a thorough interpretation. Readers should not be left to interpret statistical results without the guidance of authors.

Furthermore, Bem (2004) recommended a description of individual participants as follows:

> After you have presented your quantitative results, it is often useful to become more informal and briefly to describe the behavior of particular individuals in your study. Again, the point is not to prove something, but to add richness to your findings, to share with readers the feel of the behavior. (p. 201)

In addition, descriptions of individual subjects are helpful for transferring research to evidence-based practices. Meline and Paradiso (2003) explained the importance of individual subject descriptions to evidence-based practice as follows:

> For example, if a researcher reports a large change (for the better) between pre- and posttest means for a group of 20 subjects, does that mean that all 20 subjects improved? In reality, 10 subjects may have improved dramatically, while the remaining 10 subjects may have failed to improve at all. Thus, it is important that researchers report and interpret individual outcomes along with group results. (p. 280)

Reynolds, Callihan, and Browning (2003) asked the question: Do lessons have a significant effect on young children's rhyming skills? Reynolds et al. (2003) authored the report of an experiment that included 3- and 4-year-old children as participants. The researchers used a pretest/posttest design with participants randomly assigned to treatment and non-treatment conditions. The Reynolds et al. research team (2003) introduced their *Results section* as follows:

> An alpha level of .05 was used for all statistical tests. Results indicated a significant main effect for time; $F(1, 14) = 35.773$, $p < .05$, indicating that rhyming skills improved for all children between the pretest and the posttest. This result was qualified, however, by a significant time by group interaction, $F (1, 14) = 14.21$, $p < .05$. Examination of the mean differences in improvement for each group showed that rhyming scores improved significantly more for the experimental group (Pretest $M = 4.63$, $SD = 3.66$; Posttest $M = 16.75$, $SD = 7.68$) than they did for the control group (Pretest $M = 8.88$, $SD = 6.42$; Posttest $M = 11.63$, $SD = 8.55$). These results can be seen in Figure 1 [a line graph of pretest and posttest means]. (p. 44)

What is your evaluation of the Reynolds, et al. (2003) Results section? What information about results was included in the research report? What information is missing? How would you revise their Results section?

Writing the Discussion

The *Discussion section* is a place to evaluate and interpret the implications of the results. The APA *Publication Manual* recommends that authors open the Discussion with a statement of support or non-support for their research hypothesis. The Discussion section is also the place to comment on the importance of the findings. How do the results affect current theory? How do the results impact current practices in speech-language pathology or audiology?

Sternberg (1992) recommends that authors end the article strongly and state a clear "take-home message" for readers. Alt, Plant, and Creusere (2004) end their Discussion section with the paragraph that follows:

> The established difficulty of children with SLI in learning labels for words is paralleled in the fast-mapping of semantic features. As such, limited encoding by children with SLI has an impact on their ability to add lexical labels to their corpus of vocabulary and may lead to an impoverished understanding of the meanings conveyed by those labels acquired. Collectively, in this field, we face the challenge of discovering the exact nature of the relationship between learning lexical labels. If we are able to help children with SLI become better word learners, we need to address all components of word learning. (p. 418)

What is your evaluation of the Alt, Plante, and Creusere (2004) ending paragraph? What was their take-home message? Was it a "strong" message?

Writing the Title and Abstract

It is usually best to write the Title and Abstract after writing the Introduction, Method, Results, and Discussion sections. A title should summarize the main idea of the paper simply and with style (American Psychological Association, 2001). The title should: (a) name the variables—if possible, (b) be concise—the APA *Publication Manual* specifies 10–12 words, (c) indicate what was studied but not results or conclusions, (d) mention the population of interest if possible, and (e) use subtitles to designate the type of research—pilot study, qualitative study, or meta-analysis/synthesis study. Pyrczak and Bruce (2003) suggested including *qualitative* in the title or abstract when the study's design is qualitative. For example, Culatta, Kovarsky, Theodore, Franklin, and Timler (2003) chose the title: "Quantitative and Qualitative Documentation of Early Literacy Instruction." They also included the term *qualitative* in their abstract.

Southwood and Russell (2004) chose "Comparison of Conversation, Freeplay, and Story Generation as Methods of Language Sample Elicitation" as their research report's title. What information does the title provide? What was their research purpose? What were their experimental variables? What information is missing in the Southwood and Russell (2004) title?

Titles sometimes ask a question, though questions in titles are uncommon. Walters and Chapman (2000) asked a question in their title: "Comprehension Monitoring: A Developmental Effect?" What is your evaluation of the Walters and Chapman title? What information does the title provide? What information is missing?

Abstracts are brief, concise, and comprehensive summaries of research. The APA *Publication Manual* specifies a length of 120 words or less for abstracts. It also says that the abstract should be accurate, self-contained, non-evaluative, coherent, and readable. Furthermore, a good abstract should: (a) specify the research hypothesis, purpose, or questions, (b) provide highlights of the methodology, (c) provide highlights of the results, (d) be short, and (e) name the theory—if integral to the research. A case example is the abstract accompanying Burk and Wiley's (2004) article titled "Continuous Versus Pulsed Tones in Audiometry" as follows:

> The purpose of this study was to compare auditory thresholds obtained for continuous and pulsed tones in listeners with normal hearing. Auditory thresholds, test-retest reliability, false-positive responses, and listener preference were compared for both signals. Hearing thresholds and test-retest reliability were comparable for the 2 signals, and there were no significant differences in the number of false positives or the number of presentations required

---

Technology Note

The Internet offers many opportunities for information sharing—good and bad. Because the Internet provides access to vast archives of textual materials, papers, and articles, *plagiarism* is a potential problem. The University of Puget Sound's website—*Academic Honesty and Intellectual Ownership*—includes guidelines for academic honesty in writing along with exercises for properly citing sources.

Examples of plagiarism are included in web pages such as Princeton University's Academic Integrity site: *http://www.princeton.edu/pr/pub/integrty/pages/ plagiarism.html/*. To thwart plagiarism, plagiarism detection tools are available online—though they have limitations. *WCopyfind* is plagiarism detection freeware that compares written papers but only those files that are stored on local hard drives: *http://plagiarism.phys.virginia.edu/Wsftware.html/*. Another plagiarism detection tool, *Eve*, allows online comparisons with content published on the Internet—but not in local archives: *http://www.canexus.com/eve/index.shtml/ Turnitin.com* permits comparisons with content published on the internet and content archived in the Turnitin.com database: *http://www.turnitin.com/*.

---

to reach threshold. Listener preference, however, indicated that pulsed tones were preferred over continuous tones by 67 percent of the listeners when listening to low-level or high-frequency tones. These findings, coupled with previous reports demonstrating the benefits of using automatically pulsed tones in threshold assessment for listeners with tinnitus, support the general use of pulsed tones in clinical audiometry. (2004, p. 54)

What is your evaluation of Burk and Wiley's (2004) abstract? Does it specify the purpose? Does it provide highlights of the methodology and results? Is the abstract brief, concise, and generally readable?

Writing the References and Appendix

References appear in a list at the end of a research paper. References should account for every citation that appears in the body of the paper, including the narrative, tables, and figures. The style for writing references should follow the form specified in the APA *Publication Manual* (American Psychological Association, 2001) unless the journal's *Information for Authors* page indicates otherwise. Guidance for writing electronic citations and references is available at the American Psychological Association website: *http://www.apastyle.org/elecref.html*.

The Appendix is an optional part of the research paper but an important one. As a rule, the Appendix includes critical material that does not fit into the body of the research paper—such as samples of narratives, raw subject data, or stimulus materials.

Once a draft of the research paper is complete, the rewriting/revision stage begins. However, because the writing process is recursive and because each writer has a unique style, rewriting/revision may begin at any point in the writing/drafting stage. For example, writers may choose to write their Introduction and revise it before beginning the Method section.

The Rewriting/Revision Stage

The first draft of a research paper never achieves perfection. Authors typically encounter some serious revisions following their initial writing and first draft. Bem (2004) suggested that rewriting is especially demanding because of the following: (a) your own writing is difficult to edit, (b) rewriting requires a high degree of compulsiveness and attention to detail, and (c) substantial restructuring of the paper is usually necessary. In the latter case, rewriting typically requires authors to discard whole sections and add new ones. Some questions to consider when revising one or more sections of the research paper are as follows:

1. Is your writing sufficient in detail for a systematic replication of the study?
2. Is your writing redundant? Did you repeat unnecessary information?
3. Is your writing accurate in fact?
4. Have you cited sources of information properly?
5. Is your writing logically organized?
6. Is your interpretation of results adequate and meaningful for clinical practice?
7. Do the Method and Results support your conclusions?
8. Is your writing clear, brief, and precise?

If the answers to the preceding questions are affirmative, it is time to proceed to the editing stage. If not, authors should consider setting the paper aside for a few days or longer and returning to it later with a fresh perspective. A short break from the writing process is often helpful and usually rejuvenating.

The Editing Stage

The *editing stage* typically follows rewriting and revision, but because the writing process is recursive, editing may happen at any point in time. The use of word processors with automatic spelling and grammar checkers permits editing as writing proceeds. The editing stage has more to do with the mechanics of writing (form) and less to do with what is said (content). This is a time to make cosmetic improvements in the research paper—correct errors in spelling, punctuation, and grammar. Bem (2004) recommended the following ways to improve writing style:

1. Omit needless words.
2. Avoid meta-comments on the writing. For example, do not say, *Now that we have discussed the psychoanalytic theory of stuttering, we will explain the purpose of our experiment.*
3. Avoid jargon except when the jargon term makes an important conceptual distinction not apprehended by lay terminology.

> **Technology Note**
>
> Spell checkers, and grammar and style checking tools are useful in the editing phase of the writing process. *Microsoft Word* includes spelling and grammar checking options on its *Tools Menu,* and *WordPerfect* incorporates the *Grammatik* utility for grammar checking. The use of spell checkers is relatively free from debate; however, grammar and style checking tools are more controversial. Some English mavens warn that grammar checkers dampen creativity—students may rely on them and fail to acquire good grammar habits. Other experts argue that grammar checkers help to focus attention on sentences and constructions that may benefit from a rewrite. Clearly, grammar and style checking tools do not substitute for good writing skills, but they do help with basic writing devices such as active/passive voice, subject/verb agreement, and punctuation.

4. Use the active voice unless content dictates otherwise.
5. Use the past tense when reporting the previous research of others.
6. Avoid language bias for gender, race, sexual orientation, disabilities, and ethnicity. Guidance for *Removing Bias in Language* is available at the American Psychological Association website: *http://www.apastyle.org/elecref.html.*
7. Avoid common errors of grammar and usage. For example, the word *data* is plural, the word *none* is singular, and *that* is usually the correct relative pronoun—not *which.*

The editing stage is also a time to insure that the paper complies with writing style (usually APA) as well as other instructions found on the journal's Information for Authors page Failure to account for all the citations in the body of the research paper is a common error. The editing stage is a time for checking each citation in the body of the paper to insure that there is a corresponding reference. Furthermore, references typically contain errors of accuracy and style, so authors should carefully check references for spelling, punctuation, and form.

The Publication/Presentation Stage

Writing, rewriting, and editing tasks conclude (at least for the moment) when authors submit the research product for publication or presentation. Reviewers typically reject research papers and proposals because of one or more of the following reasons: (a) bad writing, (b) serious methodological flaws, or (c) lack of theoretical importance. Authors' diligence in rewriting and editing the paper for clarity and precision usually avoids rejection because of *bad writing.*

The most accomplished writers (and less accomplished writers) benefit from the advice of colleagues. Before submitting the research paper or proposal, authors should ask colleagues to critically read the paper and provide constructive comments. If the

> **Technology Note**
>
> Successful writing requires feedback from peers before dissemination of a paper or its submission for publication. A model for online writing help is *The Forum for Writing in Communication Sciences and Disorders*—an online writers' forum established on the University of Florida's website: *http://www.clas.ufl.edu/boards/owl/csd/*. *The Forum for Writing in Communication Sciences and Disorders* permits online comments from peers and teachers. It also allows answers to questions regarding drafts of writing assignments. Students submit their questions or writing samples and receive feedback online. The submissions to *The Forum for Writing* include literature reviews, bibliographies, resumes, and SOAP notes. To insure privacy and adhere to ethical principles, writers must redact the personal identifying information of clients, research subjects, or others before submitting written drafts for public review.

intended audience includes practitioners, authors should ask speech-language pathologists or audiologists to read the paper and share their perspectives. With colleagues' comments in hand, authors can revise the research product accordingly and submit the paper for review when they are satisfied the paper is ready.

No research product passes review without revisions. If editors do not summarily reject the paper, authors will have an opportunity to revise it. To facilitate publication, authors should carefully address reviewers' comments. Authors should submit a cover letter with the revised paper that explains how the revision incorporates the reviewers' suggestions. If authors choose not to incorporate suggestions, they should explain their rationale. The editorial process continues until editors and authors agree that the research paper is ready for publication.

CASE STUDIES

Case 12.1   Plan for Collaborative Writing?

Dr. Kroner and Ms. Parker collaborated in a research project to evaluate the efficacy of electrotherapy for treating oral/pharyngeal dysphagia. They shared equally in the planning and execution stages of the research, but Kroner and Parker are not sure who should write the research paper. They asked you for advice. What is your plan to help Kroner and Parker write their research paper?

Case 12.2   Will Julie and Eddie Avoid Plagiarism?

Julie and Eddie are students who are writing their senior theses in communication disorders. They have written their initial drafts and included content from several sources including books, journal articles, class notes, and interviews with Professors. Julie and Eddie want to avoid plagiarism, but they are not sure what content is attributable to its source—and what content does not need to be attributed to its source. They asked you for some guidance. What guidelines will you provide for Julie and Eddie?

Case 12.3   Ana and Jose Need Advice

Speech-language pathologists, Ana and Jose, are writing their research Method section, but they are not sure what to include or how much detail to include. Their study included 16 adults as participants, several commercial tests, and a set of picture cards that they designed. As the research consultant, what is your advice for Ana and Jose?

Student Exercises

1. Locate a journal article with an interesting title. Read the Abstract, evaluate its content, and identify shortcomings. Rewrite the abstract to improve its clarity and to satisfy the requirements specified in the APA *Publication Manual* (American Psychological Association, 2001).
2. Choose a research article from a communication disorders journal and evaluate its Title for content and form. Does the title meet the standards for good writing? Rewrite the title and compare your revision with the authors' title.
3. Reynolds, Callihan, and Browning (2003) reported a pretest mean and standard deviation of 4.63 (3.66) and a posttest mean and standard deviation of 16.75 (7.68). What is the effect size for their pretest/posttest results? How would you interpret the effect size?
4. Choose an article from a communication disorders journal and evaluate the Introduction's opening paragraph. Is the opening paragraph strong enough to interest readers? Does it open with a statement about people or animals? Does it include a description of the research problem? Rewrite the opening paragraph to make it stronger. HINT: Try rewriting the opening paragraph with one or more questions.
5. Choose a research report from a communication disorders journal. Evaluate the Discussion section's closing paragraph. Is the closing paragraph clear and precise? What is the authors' message in the closing paragraph? How would you rewrite the closing paragraph to improve its quality?

Evidence-Based Practice in Schools:

Evaluating Research and Reducing Barriers

TIMOTHY MELINE

The University of Texas-Pan American, Edinburg

TERI PARADISO

Brownsville Independent School District, Brownsville, TX

Abstract

This article examines the clinician/researcher relationship, suggests directions for improving the relationship, and discusses avenues for transferring information from research to clinical practice. An eight-step model for transferring research studies to practice is adopted, and three of the eight steps are targeted for discussion and illustration. To illustrate the use and interpretation of effect size measures for practical significance, as well as the transfer of research results to practice (evidence-based practice [EBP]), a case study from the contemporary literature is presented. Speech-language pathologists in schools and other work settings were surveyed to evaluate barriers to EBP. The survey suggested several possible barriers to EBP. For example, the speech-language pathologists surveyed agreed that there is not enough time on the job for research and other EBP activities. Collaborations between clinicians and researchers are recommended as a good avenue for applied research. The methods illustrated for critically evaluating research are useful for engaging EBPs. Further, clinicians in schools are encouraged to adopt EBPs with active involvement in research collaboration whenever possible.

In another paper, Meline and Mata-Pistokache (2003) wrote that "research at its best is like a Robert Ludlum novel—ingenious, thrilling, action-packed, and full of twists" (p. 3). Those words were idealized in as much as research undertakings can be tedious and research reports are sometimes boring and predictable. Meline and Wang (2002) wrote:

Reprinted by permission of the American Speech-Language-Hearing Association
Language, Speech, and Hearing Services in Schools Volume *34*, Issue 4. Pages 273–283. October 2003

The importance of research to the science of speech, language, and hearing is sometimes debated but never trivialized. Practitioners, teachers, and scientists alike depend on the body of research to further their individual goals. Practitioners seek to deliver the best services and to justify the effectiveness and efficiency of clinical services. Teachers seek knowledge to guide students in their discovery of truths or near truths. Scientists look for patterns of meaning as well as new ideas for improving the scope of knowledge in hearing, speech, and language. Speech-language pathologists and audiologists depend on research to advance the information base in speech, language, and hearing, and the information base is the heart and soul of the professions. Thus, quality of research is a matter of great importance to all. (p. 3)

It is apparent that, whether boring or exciting, research is an important part of our professional lives—clinicians, teachers, administrators, and researchers alike. Research is the foundation for the science in communication disorders, and the science is paramount to good practice.

A hot topic in communication disorders is evidence-based practice (EBP). There is much talk, numerous articles, and an abundance of presentations in local, state, and national forums about EBP. Herbert, Sherrington, Maher, and Moseley (2001) defined EBP as "the systematic use of best evidence, usually in the form of high quality clinical research, to solve clinical problems" (p. 201). Peach's (2002) editorial highlighted its importance: "Evidence-based practice is one way for clinicians to keep up-to-date with the growth in the clinical literature. It is also a means to lifelong learning and continuous improvements in one's clinical expertise" (p. 210). EBP is important because it accounts to clients, families, students in training, third-party payers, and ourselves for the use of best practices (Self & Apel, 2002).

A challenge facing clinicians in schools is to transfer research results into their practices. Law (2000) correctly noted that "the publication of research evidence in academic journals does not ensure that this information is transferred into clinical practice" (p. 33). She described a model for transferring information to practice that includes eight steps:

1. Clearly identify the clinical problem.
2. Gather information from research studies about this problem.
3. Ensure that you have adequate knowledge to read and critically analyze the research studies.
4. Decide if a research article or review is relevant to the clinical problem.
5. Summarize the information so that it can be easily used in your practice.
6. Define the expected outcomes for the children and their families.
7. Provide education and training to implement the suggested change in practice.
8. Evaluate the practice change and modify (if necessary). (pp. 33–34)

Kamhi (1999) discussed factors that influence decisions to use or not to use a new or different treatment approach. He characterized clinicians as pragmatists because they adopt therapies that work. In other words, clinicians may be more affected by observable changes in practice than by research results—what Silliman (1999) called the "seeing is knowing" phenomenon. However, Apel (1999a) argued that "without a theory, clinicians will not be able to explain why a certain cause had a specific effect" (p. 105). Nonetheless, Kazdin (2001) noted that "research can begin with variables drawn from hunches, experiences, literature, and wisdom, to mention a few sources, all of which might well be atheoretical" (p. 63). Understanding why and how therapy effects change is the ultimate goal for science; though clinicians often rely on observable changes without knowing the mechanisms of change. If the observable changes rely on the scientific method for verification (not casual observation), they are credible evidence for practice. To establish EBP, the scientific method must be adopted by clinicians as well as researchers. For example, an important scientific principle is confirmation of results. A disregard for confirmation is called confirmation bias. Tavris (2003) wrote:

> The scientific method is designed to help investigators [and clinicians] overcome the most entrenched human cognitive habit: the confirmation bias, the tendency to notice and remember evidence that confirms our beliefs or decisions, and to ignore, dismiss, or forget evidence that is discrepant. (p. B8)

In practice, confirmation bias perpetuates ideas based on confirming cases and fails to consider disconfirming cases. For example, practitioners in schools may base procedures more on their successes than on their failures. EBP requires the conscientious use of current theories, current research, and empirical data to guide practice.

The purposes of this article were to examine the clinician/researcher relationship, to recommend directions for improving the relationship, and to describe aids for transferring research to practice. The focus is on steps two, three, and four of Law's (2000) eight-step model: (a) gathering information from research studies, (b) ensuring adequate knowledge to read and analyze research studies, and (c) deciding if a research article or review is relevant to the clinical problem. However, all eight steps are important. Specifically, five questions were asked (and answers attempted):

- How should the separation between research and practice be defined?
- How should information be gathered from research studies for EBP in schools?
- What knowledge is needed to read, analyze, evaluate, and apply research to practice?
- How should decisions about relevance be made?
- How can researchers help clinicians achieve EBPs?

Research to Practice: Six Degrees of Separation?

The social psychologist, Stanley Milgram, revolutionized his field in the 1960s with ingenious but controversial experiments. In the early 1960s, he led research participants to believe that they were punishing learners with shocks (they were not). They were told to increase voltage in small increments each time a learner made a mistake on a word-matching task. Surprisingly, 65% of Milgram's participants willingly delivered shocks up to the maximum 450 volts with little hesitation. A few years later, Milgram devised an equally ingenious but less controversial experiment regarding the small world phenomenon (Milgram, 1967). Milgram gave the name, address, and some personal data for a target person (not known to subjects) who lived in Cambridge, Massachusetts, to 150 subjects in Omaha and Wichita. Subjects were told to pass the information on to a friend who was most likely to know the target person. At the experiment's conclusion, Milgram found that it took a median of five friends to reach the target person (range was 2 to 10). Thus, the notion of *six degrees of separation* was born.

How does the small world phenomenon affect research to practice? It gives promise that at the worst, there are only six degrees of separation between clinicians and researchers. At best, clinicians and researchers are separated by less than six degrees. There is also promise that e-mail, chat rooms, e-forums, and e-journals will shrink whatever degrees of separation exist between researchers and practitioners (Kuster & Poburka, 1998; Meline & Mata-Pistokache, 2003, in press). Indeed, the bridge from research to clinical practice may be shorter and sturdier than the divide envisioned by Fey and Johnson (1998).

Discussions and debates regarding the clinician/researcher relationship are not new to communication disorders. In earlier years, the separation between clinicians and researchers was described as an "artificial dichotomy" (Ringel, 1972), "dualism" (Costello, 1979), and a "dichotomy" (Schiefelbusch, 1980). Dictionary.com defines "dichotomy" as a division into two usually contradictory parts or opinions. For sure, a dichotomy (real or imagined) is unnecessary and harmful to the professions (Costello, 1979). As Costello remarked: "[A clinician/researcher dichotomy] can impede our growth of knowledge and thus ultimately effect the quality of the services we offer our clients" (1979, p. 26).

For an example of professional discord and its harm, read Tavris (2003) for her viewpoint on the clinician/researcher gap in psychology. There is much promise in reports of clinician/researcher partnerships, such as Faucheux and Oetting (2001), Goldstein and Washington (2001), and Porter and Hodson (2001). These partnerships are evidence that clinician/researcher relationships can be complementary, not contradictory. To summarize, clinicians and researchers are different in their interests and training, but they are not dichotomous. As Tavris (2003) explained: "Whenever one group is doing research and the other is working in an applied domain, their interests and training will differ" (p. B8). Fey and Johnson (1998) also observed that research and clinical practice are sometimes different endeavors, but how different are they?

Clinicians Are From Uranus, Researchers Are From Pluto

The planet Uranus is one of the largest planets in our solar system. It is also distinguished by its 18 moons. In contrast, Pluto is a small planet and is distant from the other planets. Only the most powerful telescopes are able to observe Pluto. Clinicians are many, and researchers are few. Hence, the planet Pluto and researchers are small in comparison to their counterparts. Like Uranus and its satellites, clinicians usually work at the center of constant activity. In contrast, research milieus are usually more isolated, reflective, and disconnected, somewhat like Pluto. The point is that clinicians and researchers work in distinct environments, sometimes speak different languages, and often act very differently. To paraphrase Gray (1992), when you remember that researchers are from Pluto and clinicians are from Uranus, everything can be explained. Indeed, clinicians and researchers are supposed to be different, but they should complement, not contradict, each other. Collaborative clinician/researcher efforts benefit from the differences between the two, but not without some compromise. Oetting commented: "As a researcher, I found that the most difficult aspect of this collaboration is the lack of control I had over the project" (Faucheux & Oetting, 2001).

> For individuals who are both clinicians and researchers, the dual role may present special challenges because of conflicting duties, goals, or self-interests. Sales and Lavin (2000) explained: As a scientist, the researcher's principal role-given duty is to make new discoveries, by conducting research in accordance with the best possible designs. As a therapist, the researcher's premiere [sic] role is to offer the best possible care to the participant. If therapist-researchers decide to ask clients to become participants in research, they should be cautious that they are not placing their roles as therapists and researchers in irremediable conflict because of a desire to achieve a research goal that may not be in the clients' best interest. (p. 111)

Gathering Evidence for Practice in Schools: The Five-Percent Solution?

Years ago, Fisher (1925) introduced statistical significance tests, and researchers subsequently adopted the results of analysis of variance (ANOVA) and t tests with little or no attention to the more important result, which is practical significance. Thus, the five-percent solution (i.e., reliance on the .05 level of confidence) became the standard for statistical significance. However, the five-percent solution tells us nothing about the practical significance of results, that is, the applicability and meaningfulness of results for EBP (cf. Kazdin, 1999; Meline & Schmitt, 1997; Meline & Wang, 2002). Kazdin distinguished a third kind of significance that he called clinical significance. He defined clinical significance as "the practical or applied value or importance of the effect of the intervention—that is, whether the intervention makes any real (e.g., genuine, palpable, practical, noticeable) difference in everyday life to the clients or to others with whom the client interacts" (p. 332). Thus, statistical significance is not practical significance, and practical significance may not always be clinically significant. In any case, to gather evidence for EBP, the first task is locating information and the second task is evaluating results. A discussion of these two tasks follows.

How to Locate Information for EBP

Gathering evidence for clinical practice in schools is no easy task. Once a clinical problem is clearly identified (e.g., How do I improve outcomes for children with pervasive developmental disabilities?), the next step is to find relevant information such as published research (or outcome data) about the problem. The use of search engines and the availability of online resources, such as electronic journals as well as journal archives, makes the job of gathering evidence somewhat easier. For example, the American Speech-Language-Hearing Association (ASHA) archives its journals online, and articles are available shortly after paper editions are distributed. In addition, search engines such as Google, and professional databases like ERIC and PubMed, are accessible and useful tools for locating relevant information. However, clinicians are responsible for judging the quality of the information gathered.

ASHA sponsors the National Outcomes Measurement Systems (NOMS) project, which collects information for treatment effectiveness (ASHA, n.d.). "The NOMS project, which began in 1993, is an ongoing national database of patient/client functional communication outcomes measurements" (Gallagher, 2002, p. 2). ASHA's National Center for Treatment Effectiveness in Communication Disorders developed the Functional Communication Measures (FCMs) for use in the NOMS project. The FCMs are a series of seven-point rating scales designed to measure functional progress for speech-language pathologist treatment outcomes. FCM data are collected in three components: (a) adult, (b) K-6 schools, and (c) prekindergarten. The NOMS project provides valuable outcome data for EBP. For example, based on NOMS data, ASHA reported that "[K-6] students receiving SLP services in a group setting required more treatment time than students receiving individual treatment, in order to make similar functional gains" (ASHA, n.d.).

An alternative for locating information for EBP is quality filters or prefiltered evidence. Melnyk and Fincout-Overholt (2002) explained that "prefiltered evidence means that an individual or group of individuals with expertise in a particular substantive area has reviewed and presented the methodologically strongest data in the field (Guyatt & Rennie, 2002). It includes systematic reviews as well as published evidence-based guidelines" (p. 263). A good source for systematic reviews is the meta-analyses published in mainstream journals, such as Casby's (2001) meta-analytic review for otitis media and language development. Meta-analyses are focused reviews of the research literature, but their numbers are few in speech-language pathology journals (Meline, 2003). Another source for prefiltered evidence is the Cochrane Collaboration (2003). The Cochrane Collaboration is a global network that promotes EBP. In regard to EBP guidelines, some have been developed (Academy of Neurologic Communication Disorders and Sciences, 2001), and others will be developed in the near future. The Academy of Neurologic Communication Disorders and Sciences collected and summarized evidence for practice from rigorous literature reviews. The evidence—to be disseminated as technical summaries or clinical reports—consists of practice guidelines (not standards) for making clinical decisions. Other resources for guidelines in special areas of interest, such as fluency, voice, and language, are publications by ASHA's special interest groups, such as Special Interest Division 1's newsletter, *Perspectives on Language Learning and Education*.

How to Determine if Research Reports Are Evidence for Practice

Making a decision concerning the meaningfulness of particular information to practice is no easy task. For EBP, practical significance and clinical significance are more relevant than statistical significance. The three criteria for evaluating the clinical importance of an outcome (according to Bain and Dollaghan, 1991, and reported by Meline and Schmitt, 1997) are:

- Is the change the result of treatment rather than outside variables? (internal validity)
- Is the change a real one as opposed to a random occurrence? (statistical significance)
- Is the change an important one rather than a trivial one? (practical significance)

Internal validity and practical significance are the most critical for EBP and probably the least understood.

Ruscello (1993) explained that "the concept of validity pertains to the reported observations and their adequacy in answering the research questions posed by the investigator" (p. 4). To make conclusions regarding cause and effect, a high degree of "internal validity" is essential. Internal validity has to do with the methods, procedures, and controls used by researchers. In research designs where subjects are randomly assigned to experimental and control groups, threats to internal validity are few. However, quasi-experiments are especially vulnerable because they lack randomization (Cook & Campbell, 1979). For example, randomization controls equality between groups of subjects by avoiding selection biases and maturation problems. When randomization is not possible, researchers must match subjects and adopt other controls to minimize selection biases and maturation problems. Their success or failure determines the degree of internal validity.

Though fundamentally superior to quasi-experiments, randomized experimental designs are affected by threats of another kind. For example, statistical regression, instrumentation, mortality, and testing threats affect experimental designs and quasi-experimental designs alike. Cook and Campbell (1979) outlined threats to internal validity and explained their relevance. For example, a researcher may choose subjects based on pretest scores that are extremely low. The notion of statistical regression predicts that extreme scores will increase or decrease independent of the treatment. Thus, children who evidence open syllables (final consonant deletions) 90% of the time are likely to reduce their frequencies of open syllables with or without treatment. Another threat to internal validity that affects experiments and quasi-experiments is testing (e.g., practice, learning, or fatigue). In this case, the degree of familiarity with a test may affect results independent of treatment. "When all of the threats can plausibly be eliminated, it is possible to make confident conclusions about whether a relationship is probably causal" (Cook & Campbell, 1979, p. 55).

Another important criterion for evaluating clinical significance is practical significance. The statistical measure of practical significance is called effect size (ES) (Cohen, 1988; Meline & Schmitt, 1997). Although a statistic (t or F) may be significant ($p < .05$), it may have little or no practical value. Tests of statistical significance are influenced by sample size, but effect size is not. For example, an ANOVA based on a large sample (e.g., $n = 200$) may yield a statistically significant difference between means with no practical importance. For these reasons, effect size is better evidence for clinical practice.

There are three categories for effect size statistics. The first is simple effect size. Simple effect size is the difference between treatment means. Thus, if one group of subjects is 10% disfluent and a second group is 15% disfluent, the simple effect size (difference) is 5%. However, simple effect size is only useful when the unit of measurement is familiar. In addition, simple effect size (a) does not account for variability in samples and (b) is not useful for comparing results from one study to another. A second type of effect size is the standardized effect size.[1] It resolves the shortcomings in simple effect size. Standardized effect size measures account for variation between subjects and permit comparisons between studies. A third type of effect size is the effect size correlation. For example, an effect size correlation may be computed as a point-biserial correlation between the independent variable classification and individual scores of the dependent variable. The family of correlation statistics includes Pearson r, phi, point-biserial r, and rho. Correlation statistics provide a direct index of measurement for effect size. In addition, they are easily computed from t, F, and χ^2 statistics. In the case of ANOVA, the correlation effect size is computed as $r = [\sqrt{F/F + [df_{error}]}]$ where $df = n - 1$. Though the family of standardized effect sizes (Cohen's d, Hedge's g, and Glass's $\triangle$) is more popular, some authors believe that effect size correlations are "more simply interpreted in terms of practical importance than are d or g" (Rosenthal & DiMatteo, 2001, p. 71). It may be that effect size correlations are easier to interpret because they are indexed from 0 to 1.00 (a more familiar scale). For example, equivalent values for Cohen's d and the correlation effect size are: d = 2.0 (r = .71), d = 1.5 (r = .60), d = 1.0 (r = .45), and d = 0.5 (r = .24). In practice, some researchers prefer variance-accounted-for correlation effect sizes such as r^2, R^2, and η^2. "This effect [ES^2] tells the researcher what percentage of the variability in individual differences of the participants on the outcome variable can be explained or predicted with knowledge of the group or cell membership of the participants" (Thompson, 2002a, p. 68). The prominence of effect size in ASHA journals has increased in recent years (Meline & Wang, 2002), in part because journal editors, such as Bahr (2001) and Silliman (2000), recognized its importance in their editorials.

A Case Study: Effect Size to Practice

To illustrate the use and range of interpretation for effect size (practical significance), we chose a "clinical forum" report authored by Tyler, Lewis, Haskill, and Tolbert (2002). Tyler and associates studied 27 preschoolers with language impairments—20 in an experimental group and 7 in a control group. They sought to determine and compare the effectiveness and cross-domain effects for morphosyntactic, phonologic interventions and nontreatment. The study is interesting, well conceived, and properly designed. However, as is the case with most studies, there are a few shortcomings and some potential barriers for transferring results to EBP. Tyler and associates computed standardized effect sizes for their inferential statistics (t tests), but their interpretations of effect size relied solely on Cohen's (1988) guidelines. According to Cohen's general guidelines, .20 is a small effect (small practicability), .50 is a medium effect, and .80 is a large effect. Cohen's guidelines are useful, especially when a particular behavior or phenomenon is untested. However, Cohen's guidelines should not be invoked blindly or rigidly, according to Thompson (1998, 2002a). The problem with general guidelines is that effect sizes vary from one behavior to another. Thus, effect size is dependent on the particular behavior, and general guidelines (such as Cohen's) may overestimate or underestimate true effects. If there are effect size benchmarks for a particular behavior or phenomenon, the benchmarks are the best indicators of what is a large or small effect. As Thompson (2002b) said, "The worthiness of an effect size turns largely on what one is studying" (p. 30). Once effect sizes for a particular phenomenon become normatively standard practice, clinicians are in a better position to evaluate how replicable and how stable over time a particular treatment effect may be.

One phenomenon studied by Tyler and associates (2002) was grammatical morphemes (morphosyntax), such as past tense, third-person singular, and possessive morphemes. There is a collection of research on verb morphology and grammatical morphemes, and effect sizes have typically ranged in absolute values from approximately 1.00 to 1.25 (Meline & Schmitt, 1997; Nye, Foster, & Seaman, 1987). However, effect sizes for grammatical morphemes may vary by tense relatedness (Casby & Ogiela, 2002). It seems to us (and Thompson, 1998, 2002a) that an interpretation of effect size (large, medium, or small) is better made from experience with the phenomenon at hand. In the Tyler et al. case, effect sizes that they characterized as moderately large, large, or very large may be better interpreted as typical or expected. That interpretation does not diminish the impact of their results, but it does recognize the replicability and stability of effects in the area of inquiry (morphosyntax). A seemingly important effect reported by Tyler et al. (2002) was the difference between their morphosyntax intervention group ($n = 10$) and their nontreatment control group ($n = 7$). They reported statistical significance ($p < .05$) and practical significance ($d = 1.19$). The statistic d is a standardized measure of effect size (Meline & Schmitt, 1997; Meline & Wang, 2002). Tyler and associates concluded that "a large effect size was obtained ($d = 1.19$). This speaks to the practical significance of the finding and together with statistical significance suggests the inference of treatment efficacy for the morphosyntax intervention" (p. 61). Their explanation is perfectly correct; however, there are additional ways to explain an effect size. Alternative explanations are useful because they help clinicians understand the impact of results and they ease the transfer of results to EBP. Three alternatives are depicted in Table A.1.

Table A.1 lists effect sizes, percentile standings, percentage overlap, and the chance of guessing group membership in four columns from left to right. For economy, the values

Table A.1 Alternatives for interpreting standardized effect size: (a) percentile standing, (b) percentage overlap, and (c) chance of guessing group membership.

Effect size	Percentage of subjects in control group below average subject in treated group	Percentage of overlap	Chance of guessing group membership from a single subject's score
0.0	50	100	50%
0.2	58	85	54%
0.4	66	73	58%
0.6	73	62	62%
0.8	79	53	66%
1.0	84	45	69%
1.2	88	38	73%
1.4	92	32	76%
1.6	95	27	79%
1.8	96	23	82%
2.0	98	19	84%

for effect size are abbreviated in increments from 0.0 to 2.0. Tyler and associates (2002) reported an effect size of 1.19. If that value is entered into Table A.1, an effect size of 1.19 is roughly equal to the 88th percentile in column two. Alternatively, one can say that 88% of the subjects in Tyler et al.'s control (untreated) group performed below the average subject in their morphosyntax (treated) group. A second way to explain effect size is in terms of overlap (or non-overlap) as regards a normal curve distribution. An effect size of 1.19 corresponds to a 38% overlap (see Table A.1, column 3). That means that the two groups (treated and non-treated) overlap 38%, but they differ (non-overlap) by the inverse, which is 62%. Less overlap (and more non-overlap) indicates a greater difference between groups. A third way to look at effect sizes is based on the chance (probability) of guessing group membership from one subject's performance (score). Thus, in the Tyler et al. case, their result (ES = 1.19) suggests that one will correctly guess whether a subject is a member of the group with language impairment or a member of the non-impaired group approximately 73% (nearly ¾) of the time. Finally, real-world comparisons are sometimes best for explaining the importance of an effect size because they are particularly salient. For example, an effect size of 1.0 corresponds to the average difference in height between 12- and 16-year-old boys, and Tyler et al.'s effect size is slightly greater than that value. Whatever way we choose to look at it, an effect size of 1.19 is practically significant. To evaluate *clinical significance,* clinicians will have to evaluate relevance for their own work setting, children, and other unique circumstances.

The first of several shortcomings particular to the Tyler et al. (2002) study was their interpretation (or lack of explanation) for effect sizes. A second shortcoming that is common to all group designs with small numbers of subjects is bias related to effect sizes. The problem is that studies with smaller numbers of subjects contain more sampling error. Sampling error is the difference between the sample and the larger population. All studies contain some sampling error, but it is most troublesome in the case of small samples. The effect of small samples is to create a positive bias in effect sizes (Thompson, 2002a). According to Thompson, there are three circumstances that cause positive bias for effect size: (a) studies with small sample sizes, (b) studies with more measured variables, and (c) studies conducted when the population effect size is small. In the case of small samples, there is a correction available (Thompson, 2002a). The corrected values for effect size are shrunken some and more conservative, but they are more likely to be accurate and replicable in future studies.

A third shortcoming (perhaps the most troublesome for transferring results to EBP) is lack of individual data, results, and discussion. For example, Tyler et al. (2002) reported pretreatment (baseline) data for each of the 27 subjects but did not report posttreatment data except summary statistics for groups of subjects. Without individual results, it is impossible to determine how many of their treated subjects improved and how many may not have improved. To translate research results to EBP, clinicians need individual results as well as group results and discussion. If a journal cannot expend publication space for individualized data, an online repository of results could be a valuable source of information for clinicians and researchers alike. To summarize, the Tyler et al. study is well conceived and solidly executed, with a few shortcomings that are common to many published studies.

Removing Barriers to EBP in Schools

Apel (1999b) introduced bridges from research to clinical practice in a clinical forum concerning language-learning impairments and older students in schools. Barriers to EBP might be characterized as missing planks in a bridge from research to clinical practice. What planks are missing in the bridge from research to practice? To identify barriers and recommend solutions, this section addresses four issues: (a) perceived barriers, (b) the number of researchers in communication sciences and disorders, (c) meaningful research results for practice, and (d) quality of research presentation.

Perceived Barriers to Achieving EBP

To survey speech-language pathologists concerning perceived barriers to EBP in the United States, 10 statements were borrowed from Pollock, Legg, Langhorne, and Sellars (2000) that represented three categories: ability, opportunity, and implementation (see Table A.2). To achieve a geographically diverse sample, a population of speech-language pathologists was divided into groups, and a simple random sample was drawn from each group. The groups represented five geographic regions of the United States that were identified by zip codes. ASHA's membership database was searched by zip code to identify 174 speech-language pathologists and their e-mail addresses. The aim was to poll a sufficiently large number of speech-language pathologists to conclude that the sample was representative of the population of speech-language pathologists. The survey was sent (in the body of e-mails) to the 174 addresses. Recipients were asked to identify their work settings, such as schools, hospitals, or private practices, and to agree or disagree with each of the 10 statements.

Of the 174 targeted recipients, 46 e-mails were undeliverable. A total of 30 surveys was returned, but three were unusable. The response rate for usable returns was calculated as 27/128 = 21%. The response rate and number of usable returns fell short of expectations. A minimum of 50 usable returns and a 35% response rate were expected. Because sample size determines the precision with which population values are estimated, the present sample may not represent the opinions of speech-language pathologists in general (cf. Cochran, 1977). In other words, the ability to generalize the data to the population of speech-language pathologists is limited. Of the 27 usable responses, 16 (59%) were school based, and 11 respondents were based in private practice, hospitals, agencies, rehabilitation, home health, or an unidentified work setting. The far right column in Table A.2 shows the percentage of agreement for each of the 10 statements. When only two possible outcomes (agree/disagree) exist, a special application of probability theory is useful to determine expected frequencies for combinations of outcomes. In this case, the special application is the binomial probability. A common case of binomial probability is the distribution of heads and tails following a series of coin flips. For example, if a coin is flipped 20 times and the result is 18 tails/2 heads, the outcome is interpreted as unusual and improbable. To estimate probability distributions for the present data, computer-intensive re-sampling techniques (permutation tests) were used (Good, 2000). Ten-thousand iterations for agreements and disagreements (coin flips) provided the

Table A.2   Percentage of speech-language pathologists (SLPs) agreeing with each of 10 statements.

Statements	SLPs (n = 27)
Ability	
1. I feel confident in my ability to read and understand the research literature.	96*
2. I get put off when I see statistics used in published studies.	26
Opportunity	
3. Keeping up to date with literature/research is important to me in my job.	88*
4. I am happy with the amount of time that I have available to keep up to date with literature/research.	7*
5. I share and discuss literature/research findings with the others in my department/section on a regular basis.	52
6. It is difficult to see patients and keep up to date with literature/research.	89*
Implementation	
7. I feel confident that the findings of most published research are reliable.	92*
8. I find it easy to transfer research findings into my daily practice.	42
9. The majority of literature/research that I find is not of interest to me.	44
10. There is a definite divide between research and practice.	63

*$p < .01$, two-tailed

probability distributions. For example, with 27 events (flips), 14 agreements (heads) and 13 disagreements (tails) occurred 1,514 times out of 10,000 events. This is a highly probable outcome. However, a combination of 22 heads and 5 tails occurred only 7 times in 10,000 flips—a highly improbable outcome. In this fashion, probabilities were assigned to each response in the survey. Six of the 10 responses (statements 1, 2, 3, 4, 6, and 7) were statistically improbable ($p < .01$, two-tailed).

For ability statements, nearly all (26/27) respondents expressed confidence in their ability to read and understand research literature (statement 1). Further, only approximately one in four respondents was threatened by the statistics used in published studies (statement 2). As for opportunity statements, respondents recognized the importance of keeping up to date with research (statement 3), but the group was not satisfied with the time available to read or evaluate research literature (statement 4). For implementation statements, 9 out of 10 speech-language pathologists felt confident that the findings of most published research are reliable (statement 7). The responses to the remaining four statements (5, 8, 9, and 10) were equivocal.

There are two results in the summation of data that were surprising: (a) the strong positive responses in the ability category (statements 1 and 2), and (b) the strong response to statement 7 in the implementation category. In the former case, speech-language pathologists clearly expressed confidence in their own abilities, but confidence may or may not translate to success. In the latter case, speech-language pathologists were clearly confident that most published research is reliable. That result may suggest that clinicians are not critical reviewers of research. Rather, it is possible that they accept research reports as reliable based on reputation rather than substantive review. Given the time constraints in their work places, clinicians may have little choice. Taken as a whole, the present survey suggests that speech-language pathologists want to keep up to date with the research literature, but opportunities are limited by available time. Because of sampling constraints, the results may or may not represent the opinions of speech-language pathologists as a whole.

Are There Enough Researchers in Communication Sciences and Disorders?

It is clear that the professions of speech-language pathology and audiology cannot rely on scientists/researchers in other disciplines to build our foundation of knowledge. It seems unlikely that psychologists, linguists, or others would be particularly responsive to the needs of practitioners in communication disorders. Thus, EBP depends on the willingness of our own body of researchers to address the needs of practitioners in communication disorders. The numbers of doctorate recipients in speech-language pathology and audiology varied little from 1991 to 2001. According to data from the National Opinion Research Center (NORC, n.d.), the 11-year average number of doctorates in speech-language pathology and audiology was 94, with a standard deviation of 7.5. There were three years that claimed numbers more or less than 1 SD from the average. The low was 1992, when the NORC counted 82 recipients, and the high was shared by years 1995 and 2000 (n = 106). In the most recent reporting year (2001), NORC reported 92 doctorate recipients (73 females and 19 males).

On the surface, the numbers of new doctorate recipients are good, but circumstances are troubling. The first problem is here and now, and the second problem is prospective. First, the Council of Academic Programs in Communication Sciences and Disorders (n.d.) reported that 45% to 65% of new doctorate recipients accepted college faculty positions between 1999 and 2001. In other words, nearly half of new doctorate recipients chose nonfaculty and probably non-research positions (e.g., clinical or administrative). The second problem is that of an aging college faculty and imminent retirement (or mortality). Although the economic hardships of recent years may delay retirements for some, the departures from academia may far surpass the number of new doctoral candidates in the near future. Thus, the research base that supports EBP may face hard times in future years. This is a plank in the bridge from research to practice that is particularly weak. Unless the brightest students step forward to embark on careers as researchers, the fate of EBP may be in the hands of a small cadre of researchers. A part of the solution is to involve more school clinicians in collaborative efforts with researcher/scientists. There are many examples of successful clinician/researcher partnerships, and they hold promise for more collaborations in the future (cf. Apel, 2001; Costello, 1979; Faucheux & Oetting, 2001; Goldstein & Washington, 2001).

Are Research Results and Conclusions Meaningful for Clinical Practice?

Practitioners typically work with individuals (or small groups of individuals), summarize individual performances, and write individualized reports. In contrast, researchers often work with groups of participants, summarize group performances, and write conclusions about groups of participants. It is difficult and sometimes impossible to translate results from group studies into practice when researchers report summary statistics such as means and standard deviations and ignore individual performances. Kazdin (2001) commented: "The usual focus in a study is on the gross group comparisons neglecting the question for whom change has occurred and why" (p. 65). For example, if a researcher reports a large change (for the better) between pre- and posttest means for a group of 20 subjects, does that mean that all 20 subjects improved? In reality, 10 subjects may have improved dramatically, while the remaining 10 subjects may have failed to improve at all. Thus, it is important that researchers report and interpret individual outcomes along with group results. An additional benefit is that analyzing outcomes for individuals and subgroups of individuals can help to identify different mechanisms of change (Kazdin, 2001).

Another threat to EBP is conclusion robustness. Levin (1998) said, "Conclusion robustness itself is a matter of no small concern for researchers [and practitioners], for outcome 'credibility' (Levin, 1994) and generalizability depend on it" (p. 47).

Conclusion robustness depends on the methodological adequacy of a study, including its attention to internal validity threats, external validity threats, and statistical conclusion validity. However, research studies often pass the rigor of review with inadequacies in their methodologies or faulty statistical conclusions. For example, the assumptions needed for the proper use of ANOVA may be violated (Max & Onghena, 1999). The bottom line is that clinicians cannot blindly rely on results, conclusions, and clinical recommendations in published research studies. Rather, clinicians must read and evaluate research studies with skepticism. Although quality filters are helpful tools, there is no replacement for a scientist-clinician's critical eye.

An additional problem for EBP is replication robustness. A general principle of science is that facts are not assumed until results are clearly repeated (or replicated). In other words, clinicians cannot be entirely confident that an outcome reported in a research study is meaningful until that outcome is proven to be repeatable. This is part of the confirmation process that is basic to science. To confirm results, researchers have several options. They can (a) replicate the study independently with different subjects, different sites, and different times, or (b) replicate the study by means of alternative samples of the same data from the same subjects. The latter form is internal replication, and the former is external replication. External replications are the more robust of the two kinds of replication, but either form of replication is better than none. In group research designs, researchers may use resampling techniques to confirm outcomes. Alternatively, researchers may conduct a second study with different subjects. In single-subject research designs, researchers may include additional subjects to confirm the generalizability of treatment results. Whatever the form of replication, it is important evidence of external validity for clinicians. If there is no confirmation of outcomes, clinicians should be skeptical.

Does Quality of Presentation Affect the Transfer of Research to Practice?

It would appear that authors of research reports often write for their colleagues in science instead of for clinicians in schools. In as much as clinicians are greater in number, they are a potentially larger audience for the dissemination of research findings. In a survey study, Sternberg and Gordeeva (1996) collected data to discover why some research reports are influential and others are not. They identified six factors, but the one factor that accounted for the most variation in their data was quality of presentation. Quality of presentation included items such as writing style and organization. Sternberg and Gordeeva concluded that "mere novelty is not enough. To be influential, articles have to be clearly communicated and theoretically or practically important as well" (1996, p. 75). Clearly, quality of presentation and practical significance are features that set "influential" articles apart from others. In regard to writing style, Levin (1998) argued that:

> In addition to describing what was done, how it was done, and what was found, a journal article should "tell a story." I'm not using "story" in the fictional sense here, but rather as true to life and justifiable on the basis of the study's specific operations and outcomes. Telling a story, with a clever "hook" and memorable take-home message, represents a key landmark on the publication highway (e.g., Kiewra, 1994; Levin, 1992; Sternberg, 1996). It is something that editors usually demand, reviewers seek, and readers require. (p. 50)

Indeed, an interesting writing style helps readers digest the contents of a study, generally improves readability, and makes for a more persuasive report. It would also be helpful to clinicians and researchers alike if research reports are written to satisfy the needs of both audiences. To do that, researchers must appreciate the differences that separate clinicians and researchers. To communicate better (and produce more influential articles), researchers can (a) avoid research jargon when possible and provide explanations in a clinical vernacular; (b) form results and conclusions that are meaningful for practice in schools; and (c) provide data, graphs, analyses, and the like for individual subjects as well as for groups of subjects.

It seems clear that school practitioners are able participants in the research to practice process. At the least, clinicians can gain expert skills, specialize in areas of interest, and share information with colleagues to advance their EBPs. At the most, clinicians can engage in applied research activities with research/scientist mentors, collaborators, or colleagues. However, is it possible that clinicians in schools may be dressed in their best EBP garb with no place to go?

All Dressed up and No Place to Go?

Bennett (1993) asked the question: Are teacher-researchers all dressed up with no place to go? Bennett surveyed teachers in schools and discovered significant benefits for teachers who learned to apply research in their classrooms. According to Bennett: "[Teachers] saw little value in educational research and made no connection between research and effective classroom practice" (1993, p. 69). However, experienced teacher-researchers "viewed themselves as being more open to change, more reflective, and better informed than they had been when they began their research" (Bennett, 1993, p. 69). Bennett added, "They also saw a strong connection between theory and practice" (1993, p. 69). These remarks are testaments to the value of research in practice. These statements would suggest that whatever the level of participation, clinicians in schools benefit dramatically from research. However, the problem is that "for [clinician-researchers] to contribute to educational change, they need school and district support for their new roles" (Bennett, 1993, p. 69). It seems that a significant barrier for many clinicians in schools is adequate time for research and other EBP activities.

To summarize, five questions were addressed:

- How should the separation between research and practice be defined?
- How should information be gathered from research studies for EBP in schools?
- What knowledge is needed to read, analyze, evaluate, and apply research to practice?
- How should decisions about relevance be made?
- How can researchers help clinicians achieve EBPs?

Each question was addressed in turn. To that end, the authors' opinions were shared in a dual effort: (a) to persuade clinicians and researchers to better appreciate the differences that separate the two endeavors, and (b) to persuade clinicians to adopt sound research principles and critically review research. For readers who wish to compute effect sizes from the inferential statistics (e.g., F and t) reported in published research articles, Lyons (2002) offers a meta-analysis calculator as freeware at his web site. It requires a few simple entries, and effect sizes are readily computed.

The dynamic of the clinician/researcher relationship is give and take. No individual or group has a lock on good ideas. Rather, both researchers and clinicians possess unique skills and experiences that are enhanced when they are combined in collaborative efforts. Both clinicians and researchers must overcome serious obstacles before EBP is realized at its best. However, this is no mission impossible.

References

Academy of Neurologic Communication Disorders and Sciences, (2001, August). Evidence-based practice guidelines for the management of communication disorders in neurologically impaired individuals: Project introduction.

American Speech-Language-Hearing Association, Resource Center: National Outcomes Measurement System, (n.d.). National Center for Treatment Effectiveness in Communication Disorders.

Apel, K. (1999a). Checks and balances: Keeping the science in our profession. *Language, Speech, and Hearing Services in Schools. 30.* 98–107.

Apel, K. (1999b). An introduction to assessment and intervention with older students with language-learning impairments: Bridges from research to clinical practice. *Language, Speech, and Hearing Services in Schools. 30.* 228–230.

Apel, K. (2001). Developing evidence-based practices and research collaborations in school settings. *Language, Speech, and Hearing Services in Schools. 32.* 149–152.

Bahr, R. H. (2001). From the editor. *Language, Speech, and Hearing Services in Schools. 32.* 3.

Bain, B. A., & Dollaghan, C. A. (1991). The notion of clinically significant change. *Language, Speech, and Hearing Services in Schools. 22.* 264–270.

Bennett, C. K. (1993). Teacher-researchers: All dressed up and no place to go?. *Educational Leadership. 51.* 69–70.

Bird, K. D. (2002). Confidence intervals for effect sizes in analysis of variance. *Educational and Psychological Measurement. 62.* 197–226.

Casby, M. W. (2001). Otitis media and language development: A meta-analysis. *American Journal of Speech-Language Pathology. 10.* 65–80.

Casby, M. W., & Ogiela, D. (2002, November). Grammatical morphology and specific language impairment: A meta-analysis. Poster session presented at the annual meeting of the American Speech-Language-Hearing Association, Atlanta, GA.

Cochran, W. G. (1977). *Sampling techniques.* New York: John Wiley & Sons. Cochrane Collaboration, (2003). US Cochrane Center.

Cohen, J. (1988). *Statistical power analysis for the behavioral sciences.* Hillsdale, NJ: Lawrence Erlbaum & Associates.

Cook, T. D., & Campbell, D. T. (1979). *Quasi-experimentation: Design and analysis issues for field settings.* Boston: Houghton Mifflin.

Costello, J. M. (1979). Clinician and researchers: A necessary dichotomy? *Journal of the National Student Speech and Hearing Association, 7,* 6–26.

Council of Academic Programs in Communication Sciences and Disorders, (n.d.). 2000–01 demographic survey of undergraduate and graduate programs in communication sciences and disorders.

Cumming, G. (2001). Exploratory software for confidence intervals [Computer software]. Bundoora: La Trobe University.

Cumming, G., & Finch, S. (2001). A primer on the understanding, use, and calculation of confidence intervals that are based on central and noncentral distributions. *Educational and Psychological Measurement. 61.* 532–574.

Faucheux, S., & Oetting, J. (2001, October 9). A clinician-researcher partnership: Working together to improve academic services in middle school. *The ASHA Leader, 6,* 4–5, 17.

Fey, M. E., & Johnson, B. W. (1998). Research to practice (and back again) in speech-language intervention. *Topics in Language Disorders. 18.* 23–34.

Fidler, F., & Thompson, B. (2001). Computing correct confidence intervals for ANOVA fixed- and random-effects effect sizes. *Educational and Psychological Measurement. 61.* 575–604.

Fisher, R. A. (1925). Statistical methods for research workers. Edinburgh: Oliver & Boyd.

Gallagher, T. M. (2002). Evidence-based practice: Applications to speech-language pathology. *Perspectives on Language Learning and Education. 9.* 2–5.

Goldstein, B., & Washington, P. S. (2001). An initial investigation of phonological patterns in typically developing 4-year-old Spanish-English bilingual children. *Language, Speech, and Hearing Services in Schools. 32.* 153–164.

Good, P. (2000). *Permutation tests: A practical guide to resampling methods for testing hypotheses.* New York: Springer.

Gray, J. (1992). *Men are from Mars, women are from Venus: A practical guide for improving communication and getting what you want in your relationships.* New York: Harper Collins.

Guyatt, G., & Rennie, D. (2002). *Users' guides to the medical literature. Essentials of evidence-based clinical practice.* Chicago: AMA Press.

Herbert, R. D., Sherrington, C., Maher, C., & Moseley, A. M. (2001). Evidence-based practice-imperfect but necessary. *Physiotherapy Theory and Practice. 17.* 201–211.

Kamhi, A. G. (1999). To use or not use: Factors that influence the selection of new treatment approaches. *Language, Speech, and Hearing Services in Schools. 30.* 92–98.

Kazdin, A. E. (1999). The meanings and measurement of clinical significance. *Journal of Consulting and Clinical Psychology. 67.* 332–339.

Kazdin, A. E. (2001). Bridging the enormous gaps of theory with therapy research and practice. *Journal of Clinical Child Psychology. 30.* 59–66.

Kiewra, K. A. (1994). A slice of advice. *Educational Researcher. 23.* 31–33.

Kuster, J. M., & Poburka, B. J. (1998). The Internet: A bridge between research and practice. *Topics in Language Disorders. 18.* 71–87.

Law, M. (2000). Strategies for implementing evidence-based practice in early intervention. *Infants and Young Children. 13.* 32–40.

Levin, J. R. (1992). Tips for publishing and professional writing. *Mid-Western Educational Researcher. 5.* 12–14.

Levin, J. R. (1994). Crafting educational intervention research that's both credible and creditable. *Educational Psychology Review. 6.* 231–243.

Levin, J. R. (1998). What if there were no more bickering about statistical significance tests? *Research in the Schools. 5.* 43–53.

Lyons, L. C. (2002). Meta-analysis calculator [Computer software].

Max, L., & Onghena, P. (1999). Some issues in the statistical analysis of completely randomized and repeated measures designs for speech, language, and hearing research. *Journal of Speech, Language, and Hearing Research. 42.* 261–270.

Meline, T. (2003). Publication bias in meta-analysis: Fact or fiction? Manuscript submitted for publication.

Meline, T., & Mata-Pistokache, T. (2003). From paper to cyberspace: Where does the chain of publication end?

Meline, T., & Mata-Pistokache, T. (in press) The perils of Pauline's e-mail: Professional issues for audiologists and speech-language pathologists. *Contemporary Issues in Communication Science and Disorders.*

Meline, T., & Schmitt, J. F. (1997). Case studies for evaluating significance in group designs. *American Journal of Speech-Language Pathology. 6.* 33–41.

Meline, T., & Wang, B. (2002). Effect-size reporting practices in AJSLP and other ASHA journals 1997–2001. Manuscript submitted for Publication.

Melnyk, B. M., & Fincout-Overholt, E. (2002). Key steps in implementing evidence-based practice: Asking compelling, searchable questions and searching for the best evidence. *Pediatric Nursing. 22.* 262–263, 266.

Milgram, S. (1967). The small world problem. *Psychology Today. 1.* 60–67.

National Opinion Research Center, (n.d.). Doctorate recipients from United States universities: Summary report 2001.

Nye, C., Foster, S. H., & Seaman, D. (1987). Effectiveness of language intervention with the language/learning disabled. *Journal of Speech and Hearing Research. 36.* 1249–1257.

Peach, R. K. (2002). From the editor. *American Journal of Speech-Language Pathology. 11.* 210.

Pollock, A. S., Legg, L., Langhorne, P., & Sellars, C. (2000). Barriers to achieving evidence-based stroke rehabilitation. *Clinical Rehabilitation. 14.* 611–617.

Porter, J. H., & Hodson, B. W. (2001). Collaborating to obtain phonological acquisition data for local schools. *Language, Speech, and Hearing Services in Schools. 32.* 165–171.

Ringel, R. L. (1972, July). The clinician and the researcher: An artificial dichotomy. *Asha. 14.* 351–353.

Rosenthal, R., & DiMatteo, M. R (2001). Meta-analysis: Recent developments in quantitative methods for literature reviews. *Annual Review of Psychology. 52.* 59–82.

Ruscello, D. M. (1993). Evaluating research for clinical practice: A guide for practitioners. *Clinics in Communication Disorders. 3.* 1–8.

Sales, B. D., & Lavin, M. (2000). Identifying conflicts of interest and resolving ethical dilemmas. Ethics in research with human participants. Washington, DC: American Psychological Association. pp. 109–128.

Schiefelbusch, R. L. (1980, October). The role of science in speech-language pathology and audiology. *Asha. 22.* 906–908.

Schmidt, F., & Hunter, J. E. (1995). The impact of data-analysis methods on cumulative research knowledge: Statistical significance testing, confidence intervals, and meta-analysis. *Evaluation and the Health Professions. 18.* 408–427.

Schmidt, F. L. (1996). Statistical significance testing and cumulative knowledge in psychology: Implications for training of researchers. *Psychological Methods. 1.* 115–129.

Self, T., & Apel, K. (2002, November). Evidenced-based practices: Backing up clinical services with research. Paper presented at the annual meeting of the American Speech-Language-Hearing Association, Atlanta, GA.

Silliman, E. R. (1999). From the editor. *Language, Speech, and Hearing Services in Schools. 30.* 131.

Silliman, E. R. (2000). From the editor. *Language, Speech, and Hearing Services in Schools. 31.* 115.

Smithson, M. (2001). Correct confidence intervals for various regression effect sizes and parameters: The importance of noncentral distributions in computing intervals. *Educational and Psychological Measurement. 61.* 605–632.

Sternberg, R. J. (1996). *The psychologist's companion: A guide to scientific writing for students and researchers.* Cambridge: Cambridge University Press.

Sternberg, R. J., & Gordeeva, T. (1996). The anatomy of impact: What makes an article influential? *Psychological Science. 8.* 69–75.

Tavris, C. (2003, February). Mind games: Psychological warfare between therapists and scientists. *The Chronicle Review. 49.* B7–B9.

Thompson, B. (1998, April). Five methodology errors in educational research: The pantheon of statistical significance and other faux pas. Invited address presented at the meeting of the American Educational Research Association, San Diego, CA.

Thompson, B. (2002a). "Statistical," "practical," and "clinical": How many kinds of significance do counselors need to consider? *Journal of Counseling and Development. 80.* 64–71.

Thompson, B. (2002b). What future quantitative social science research could look like: Confidence intervals for effect sizes. *Educational Researcher. 31.* 25–32.

Tyler, A. A., Lewis, K. E., Haskill, A., & Tolbert, L. C. (2002). Efficacy and cross-domain effects of a morphosyntax and a phonology intervention. *Language, Speech, and Hearing Services in Schools. 33.* 52–66.

Footnotes

[1] A discussion of confidence intervals and their non-central distributions for effect size is omitted because the topic is specialized and thoroughly explained elsewhere (cf. Bird, 2002; Cumming, 2001; Cumming & Finch, 2001; Fidler & Thompson, 2001; Schmidt, 1996; Schmidt & Hunter, 1995; Smithson, 2001).

BIBLIOGRAPHY

Abraham, S., & Stoker, R. (1988). Language assessment of hearing–impaired children and youth: Patterns of test use. *Language, Speech, and Hearing Services in Schools, 19,* 160–174.

Academic Writing for Publication, (2002). Retrieved August 27, 2004, from Hong Kong Polytechnic University, The Department of English Web site: *http://www.engl.polyu.edu.hk/EECTR/awphandbook/AWP.htm*

AllPsych ONLINE, (2004). *The virtual psychology classroom.* Retrieved August 27, 2004 from *http://allpsych.com*

Almer, E. C. (2000). *Statistical tricks and traps: An illustrated guide to the misuses of statistics.* Los Angeles: Pyrczak Publishing.

Alt, M., Plante, E., & Creusere, M. (2004). Semantic features in fast–mapping: performance of preschoolers with specific language impairment versus preschoolers with normal language. *Journal of Speech–Language–Hearing Research, 47,* 407–420.

Ambrose, N. G., & Yairi, E. (2002). The Tudor study: Data and ethics. *American Journal of Speech–Language Pathology, 11,* 190–203.

American Academy of Audiology, (2004a). *Code of ethics & procedures, rules & penalties.* Retrieved August 27, 2004 from, *http://www.audiology.org /about/code.pdf*

American Academy of Audiology, (2004b). *Publications.* Retrieved August 29, 2004 from, *http://www.audiology.org/professional/pubs/*

American Psychological Association, (2001). *Publication manual of the American psychological association.* Washington: Author.

American Psychological Association, (2002). *Ethical principles of psychologists and code of conduct.* Retrieved August 26, 2004 from, *http://www.apa.org/ethics/code2002.html*

American Speech–Language–Hearing Association, (1994). The role of research and the state of research training within communication sciences and disorders. *Asha, 36* (March, Suppl. 12), 21–23.

American Speech–Language–Hearing Association, (2003). Code of ethics (revised). *ASHA Supplement, 25,* 13–15.

American Speech–Language–Hearing Association, (2004). *ASHA publications.* Retrieved August 29, 2004 from, *http://www.asha.org/about/publications*

Amlani, A. M. (2001). Efficacy of directional microphone hearing aids: A meta–analytic perspective. *Journal of the American Academy of Audiology, 12,* 202–214.

Andrews, G., Guitar, B., & Howie, P. (1980). Meta–analysis of the effects of stuttering treatment. *Journal of Speech and Hearing Disorders, 45,* 287–307.

Association of College and Research Libraries, (2000). *ACRL Information Literacy Web Site.* Retrieved August 27, 2004 from, *http://www.ala.org.*

Beeman, S. K. (2002). *Evaluating violence against women research reports.* Applied Research Forum: National Electronic NetWork on Violence Against Women. Retrieved August 27, 2004 from, *http://www.vawnet.org/DomesticViolence/Research/vawnetDocs/ AR_evalresearch.PDF*

Bem, D. J. (2004). Writing the empirical article. In J. M. Darley, M. P. Zanna, & H. L. Roediger III (Eds.), *The compleat academic: A career guide* (pp. 185–219). Washington, DC: American Psychological Association.

Bender, B. K., Cannito, M. P., Murray, T., & Woodson, G. E. (2004). Speech intelligibility in severe adductor spasmodic dysphonia. *Journal of Speech–Language–Hearing Research, 47,* 21–32.

Berlin, J. A., Laird, N. M., Sacks, H. S., & Chalmers, T. C. (1989). A comparison of statistical methods for combining event rates from clinical trials. *Statistics in Medicine, 8,* 141–151.

Black, N. (1996). Why we need observational studies to evaluate the effectiveness of health care. *BMJ, 312,* 1215–1218.

Bloom, L. (1970). *Language development: Form and function in emerging grammars.* Cambridge, MA: The M.I.T. Press.

Blood, G. W., Ridenour, J. S., Thomas, E. A., Qualls, C. D., & Hammer, C. S. (2002). Predicting job satisfaction among speech–language pathologists working in public schools. *Language, Speech, and Hearing Services in Schools, 33,* 282–290.

Bok, S. (1999). *Lying: Moral choice in public and private life.* New York: Vintage Books.

Borden, G. J., Harris, K. S., & Raphael, L. J. (2002). *Speech science primer: Physiology, acoustics, and perception of speech.* New York: Lippincott Williams & Wilkins.

Boutsen, F., Cannito, M. P., Taylor, M., & Bender, B. (2002). Botox treatment in adductor spasmodic dysphonia: A meta–analysis. *Journal of Speech–Language–Hearing Research, 45,* 469–481.

Bracht, G. H., & Glass, G. V. (1968). The external validity of experiments. *American Educational Research Journal, 5,* 437–474.

Brobeck, T. C., & Lubinsky, J. (2003). Using single–subject designs in speech–language pathology practicum. *Contemporary Issues in Communication Science and Disorders, 30,* 101–106.

Brookshire, R. H. (1983). Subject description and generality of results in experiments with aphasic adults. *Journal of Speech and Hearing Disorders, 48,* 342–346.

Burk, M. H., & Wiley, T. L. (2004). Continuous versus pulsed tones in audiometry. *American Journal of Audiology, 13,* 54–61.

California Employment Development Department, (1995). *California occupational guide number 453.* Retrieved August 26, 2004 from, *http://www.calmis.cahwnet.gov/file/occguide/SPEECHPA.HTM*

Campbell, J. P. (1982). Editorial: Some remarks from the outgoing editor. *Journal of Applied Psychology, 67,* 691–700.

Campbell, D. T. (1957). Factors relevant to the validity of experiments in social settings. *Psychological Bulletin, 54,* 297–312.

Campbell, D. T., & Stanley, J. C. (1963). Experimental and quasi–experimental designs for research or teaching. In N. L. Gage (Ed.), *Handbook of Research on Teaching* (pp. 171–246) Chicago: Rand McNally.

Cannito, M. P. & Kondraske, G. V. (1990). Rapid manual abilities in spasmodic dysphonic and normal female subjects. *Journal of Speech and Hearing Research, 33,* 123–133.

Carr, J. E., & Burkholder, E. O. (1998). Creating single–subject design graphs with Microsoft EXCEL. *Journal of Applied Behavior Analysis, 31,* 245–251.

Carrow–Woolfolk, E. (1999). *Test of auditory comprehension of language (TACL 3).* Circle Pines, MN: AGS Publishing.

Casby, M. W. (2001). Otitis media and language development: A meta–analysis. *American Journal of Speech–Language Pathology, 10,* 65–80.

Catts, H. W., Fey, M. E., Tomblin, J. B., & Zhang, X. (2002). A longitudinal investigation of reading outcomes in children with language impairments. *Journal of Speech–Language–Hearing Research, 45,* 1142–1157.

Chambers, J. M., Cleveland, W. S., Kleiner, B., & Tukey, P. A. (1983). *Graphical methods for data analysis.* Belmont, CA: Wadsworth.

Collins, C. R., & Blood, G. W. (1990). Acknowledgement and severity of stuttering as factors influencing nonstutterers' perceptions of stutterers. *Journal of Speech and Hearing Disorders, 55,* 75–81.

Condouris, K., Meyer, E., & Tager–Flusberg, H. (2003). The relationship between standardized measures of language and measures of spontaneous speech in children with autism.

American Journal of Speech–Language Pathology, 13, 349–358.

Court of Appeals of Maryland, (2001). *Ericka Grimes* v. *Kennedy Krieger Institute, Inc. (No. 128) case number 24–C–99–000925*. Retrieved August 27, 2004 from, *http://www.courts.state .md.us/opinions/coa/2001/128a00.pdf*

Cox, L. R., Cooper, W. A., & McDade, H. L. (1989). Teachers' perceptions of adolescent girls who wear hearing aids. *Language, Speech, and Hearing Services in Schools, 20,* 372–380.

Cox, K. M., Lee, D. J., Carey, J. P., & Minor, L. B. (2003). Dehiscence of bone overlying the superior semicircular canal as a cause of an air–bone gap on audiometry: A case study. *American Journal of Audiology, 12,* 11–6.

Cream, A., Onslow, M., Packman, A., and Llewellyn, G. (2003). Protection from harm: The experience of adults after therapy with prolonged speech. *International Journal of Language and Communication Disorders, 38,* 379–395.

Crosbie, J. (1993). Interrupted time series analysis with brief single–subject data. *Journal of Consulting and Clinical Psychology, 61,* 966–974.

Culatta, B., Kovarsky, D., Theadore, G., Franklin, A., & Timler, G. (2003). Quantitative and qualitative documentation of early literacy instruction. *American Journal of Speech–Language Pathology, 12,* 173–188.

Damico, J. S., & Simmons–Mackie, N. N. (2003). Qualitative research and speech–language pathology: A tutorial for the clinical realm. *American Journal of Speech–Language Pathology, 12,* 131–143.

Daniels, S. K., Corey, O. M., Hodskey, L. D., Legendre, C., Priestly, D. H., Rosenbeck, J. C., & Foundas, A. L. (2004). Mechanism of sequential swallowing during straw drinking in healthy young and older adults. *Journal of Speech–Language–Hearing Research, 47,* 33–45.

Dekroon, D. M. A., Kyle, C. S., & Johnson, C. J. (2002). Partner influences on the social pretend play of children with language impair-ments. *Language, Speech, and Hearing Services in Schools, 33,* 253–267.

DePaul, R., & Kent, R. D. (2000). A longitudinal case study of ALS: Effects of listener familiarity and proficiency on intelligibility judgments. *American Journal of Speech–Language Pathology, 9,* 230–240.

Digital Era Copyright Enhancement Act, (1999). Retrieved August 26,2004 from, *http://www .copyright.gov*.

Dunn, L. M., & Dunn, L. M. (1997). *Peabody picture vocabulary test (PPVT 3)*. Circle Pines, MN: AGS Publishing.

Eadie, P. A., Fey, M. E., Douglas, J. M., & Parsons, C. L. (2002). Profiles of grammatical morphology and sentence imitation in children with specific language impairment and Down syndrome. *Journal of Speech–Language–Hearing Research, 45,* 720–732.

Egger, M., Schneider, M., Smith, G. D. (1998). Meta–analysis: Spurious precision? Meta–analysis of observational studies. *BMJ, 316,* 140–144.

Egger, M., & Smith, G. D. (1997). Meta–analysis: Potentials and promise. *BMJ, 315,* 1371–1374.

Egger, M., Smith, G. D., & Phillips, A. N. (1997). Meta–analysis: Principles and procedures. *BMJ, 315,* 1533–1537.

Egger, M., Smith, G. D., Schneider, M., & Minder, C. (1997). Bias in meta–analysis detected by a simple graphical test. *BMJ, 315,* 629–634.

Eisenberg, S. L., Fersko, T. M., & Lundgren, C. (2001). The use of MLU for identifying language impairment in preschool children: A review. *American Journal of Speech–Language Pathology, 10,* 323–342.

Ekman, P., & Friesen, W. V. (1969). The repertoire of nonverbal behavior: Categories, origins, usage, and coding. *Semiotica, 1,* 49–98.

Emanuel, D. C. (2002). The auditory processing battery: Survey of common practices. *Journal of the American Academy of Audiology, 13,* 93–117.

Emig, J. A. (1971). *The composing processes of twelfth graders*. Urbana, IL: The National Council of Teachers of English.

Erler, S. F., & Garstecki, D. C. (2002). Hearing loss-and hearing aid-related stigma: Perceptions of women with age–normal hearing. *American Journal of Audiology, 11,* 83–91.

Ethics Board (2002). *Ethics in research and professional practice.* Retrieved August 27, 2004 from, *http://www.asha.org/NR/rdonlyres/750A 8380-D6CD-4591-97E7-C4E794A665DB/0/ 18792_1.pdf.*

Eysenbach, G. & Till, J. E. (2001). Ethical issues in qualitative research on internet communities. *BMJ, 323,* 1103–1105.

Faith, M. S., Allison, D. B., & Gorman, B. S. (1997). Meta–analysis of single–case research. In Franklin, R. D., Allison, D. B., & Gorman, B. S. (Eds.), Design and Analysis of Single-Case Research (pp. 245–277). Mahwah, NJ: Lawrence Erlbaum.

Flower, L., & Hayes, J. R. (1981). A cognitive process theory of writing. *College Composition and Communication, 32,* 365–387.

Franklin, R. D., Allison, D. B., & Gorman, B. S. (1997). Design and analysis of single–case research. Mahwah, NJ: Lawrence Erlbaum.

Frazek, M. (2003). Ethics vs. legal jurisdiction. *ASHA LeaderOnline.* Retrieved August 29, 2004 from, *http://www.asha.org/about/ethics/ ethics-jurisdiction.htm.*

Freund, J. E. (1988). *Modern elementary statistics.* Englewood Cliffs, NJ: Prentice–Hall.

Friedman, M. I. (1953). *Essays in positive economics.* Chicago: University of Chicago Press.

Gelfand, S. A., Schwander, T., & Silman, S. (1990). Acoustic reflex thresholds in normal and cochlear–impaired ears: Effects of no–response rates on 90th percentiles in a large sample. *Journal of Speech and Hearing Disorders, 55,* 198–205.

Gibbs, G. R., Friese, S., & Mangabeira, W. C. (2002, May). The use of new technology in qualitative research. *Using Technology in the Qualitative Research Process, 3,* No. 2. Retrieved August 27, 2004 from, *http://www .qualitative-research.net/fqs-texte/2-02/2-02 hrsg-e.htm*

Girden, E. R. (1996). *Evaluating research articles from start to finish.* Thousand Oaks, CA: Sage.

Glennen, S. (2002). Language development and delay in internationally adopted infants and toddlers: A review. *American Journal of Speech–Language Pathology, 11,* 333–339.

Goldstein, B., & Washington, P. S. (2001). An initial investigation of phonological patterns in typically developing 4 year–old Spanish–English bilingual children. *Language, Speech, and Hearing Services in Schools, 32,* 153–164.

GraphPad Quick Calcs, (2004). *Free online calculators for scientists.* Retrieved August 26, 2004 from, *http://www.graphpad.com*

Green, J., & Britten, N. (1998). Qualitative research and evidence based medicine. *BMJ, 316,* 1230–1232.

Greenhalgh, T. (1997a). How to read a paper: The Medline database. *BMJ, 315,* 180–183.

Greenhalgh, T. (1997b). How to read a paper: Papers that summarize other papers (systematic reviews and meta–analyses). *BMJ, 315,* 672–675.

Greenhalgh, T. (1998). Outside the ivory towers: Evidence based medicine in the real world. *The British Journal of General Medicine, 48,* 1448–1449.

Greenhalgh, T. (2001). *How to read a paper: The basics of evidence based medicine.* London: BMJ Books.

Grose, J. H., Hall III, J. W., & Bass, E. (2004). Duration discrimination in listeners with cochlear hearing loss: Effects of stimulus type and frequency. *Journal of Speech–Language–Hearing Research, 47,* 5–12.

Guitar, B., & Marchinkoski, L. (2001). Influence of mothers' slower speech on their children's speech rate. *Journal of Speech–Language–Hearing Research, 44,* 853–861.

Guyatt, G., Jaeschke, R., Heddle, N., Cook, D., Shannon, H., & Walter, S. (1995). Basic statistics for clinicians 1: Hypothesis testing. *Canadian Medical Association Journal, 152,* 27–32.

Hedges, L. V., Gurevitch, J., & Curtis, P. S. (1999). The meta–analysis of response ratios in experimental ecology: Meta–analysis in ecology. *Ecology, 80,* 1150–1156.

Hedges, L. V., & Olkin, I. (1985). *Statistical methods for meta–analysis.* San Diego, CA: Academic Press.

Herbert, R. D., Sherrington, C., Maher, C., & Moseley, A. M. (2001). Evidence–based practice–imperfect but necessary. *Physiotherapy Theory and Practice, 17,* 201–211.

Hersen, M., & Barlow, D. H. (1976). *Single case experimental designs: Strategies for studying behavior change.* New York: Pergamon Press.

Hetzroni, O. E., Quist, R. W., & Lloyd, L. L. (2002). Translucency and complexity: Effects on Bliss-symbol learning using computer and teacher presentations. *Language, Speech, and Hearing Services in Schools, 33,* 291–303.

Hinkle, D. E., Wiersma, W., & Jurs, S. G. (1988). *Applied statistics for the behavioral sciences.* Boston: Houghton Mifflin.

Hoffman, V., & Gillam, R. R. (2004). Verbal and spatial information processing constraints in children with specific language impairment. *Journal of Speech–Language–Hearing Research, 47,* 114–125.

Holcomb, Z. C. (2004). *Interpreting basic statistics.* Glendale, CA: Pyrczak Publishing.

Hopper, T., Bayles, K. A., Harris, F. P., & Holland, A. (2001). The relationship between minimum data set ratings and scores on measures of communication and hearing among nursing home residents with dementia. *American Journal of Speech–Language Pathology, 10,* 370–381.

Hubbard, C. P. (1998). Stuttering, stressed syllables, and word onsets. *Journal of Speech–Language–Hearing Research, 41,* 802–808.

Huer, M. B., & Saenz, T. I. (2003). Challenges and strategies for conducting survey and focus group research with culturally diverse groups. *American Journal of Speech–Language Pathology, 12,* 209–220.

Ingham, R. J., Fox, P. T., Ingham, J. C., Xiong, J., Zamarripa, F., Hardies, L. J., & Lancaster, J. L. (2004). Brain correlates of stuttering and syllable production: Gender comparison and

replication. *Journal of Speech–Language–Hearing Research, 47,* 321–341.

Jarvis, L. H., Merriman, W. E., Barnett, M., Hanba, J., & Van Haitsma, K. S. (2004). Input that contradicts young children's strategy for mapping novel words affects their phonological and semantic interpretation of other novel words. *Journal of Speech–Language–Hearing Research, 47,* 392–406.

Jupiter, T., & Palagonia, C. L. (2001). The hearing handicap inventory for the elderly screening version adapted for use with elderly Chinese American individuals. *American Journal of Audiology, 10,* 99–103.

Justice, L. M., Chow, Sy–Min, Capellini, C., Flanigan, K., & Colton, S. (2003). Emergent literacy intervention for vulnerable preschoolers: Relative effects of two approaches. *American Journal of Speech–Language Pathology, 12,* 320–332.

Justice, L. M., Weber, S. E., Ezell, H. K., & Bakeman, R. (2002). A sequential analysis of children's responsiveness to parental print references during shared book-reading interactions. *American Journal of Speech–Language Pathology, 11,* 30–40.

Kamhi, A. G. (2004). A meme's eye view of speech-language pathology. *Language, Speech, and Hearing Services in Schools, 35,* 105–111.

Kavale, K. A. (2001). Meta–analysis: A primer. *Exceptionality, 9,* 177–183.

Kazdin, A. E. (1982). Single–case experimental designs. In P. C. Kendall & J. N. Butler (Eds.), *Handbook of Research Methods in Clinical Psychology* (pp. 461–490). Hoboken, NJ: John Wiley & Sons.

Kerlinger, F. N. (1973). *Foundations of behavioral research.* New York: Holt, Rinehart and Winston.

Kerlinger, F. N. (1979). *Behavioral research: A conceptual approach.* New York: Holt, Rinehart and Winston.

Keselman, H. J., Huberty, C. J., Lix, L. M., Olejnik, S., Cribbie, R. A., Donahue, B., Kowalchak, R. K., Lowaman, L. L., Petoskey, M. D., & Keselman, J. C. (1998). Statistical practices of educational researchers: An analysis of their

ANOVA, MANOVA, and ANCOVA analyses. *Review of Educational Research, 68,* 350–386.

Kiran, S., & Thompson, C. K. (2003). The role of semantic complexity in treatment of naming deficits: Training semantic categories in fluent aphasia by controlling exemplar typicality. *Journal of Speech–Language–Hearing Research, 46,* 608–622.

Korchin, S. J., & Cowan, P. A. (1982). Ethical perspectives in clinical research. In P. C. Kendall & J. N. Butcher (Eds.). *Handbook of Research Methods in Clinical Psychology* (pp. 59–94). New York: John Wiley & Sons.

Kratochwill, T. R. (1978). *Single subject research: Strategies for evaluating change.* New York: Academic Press.

Kritikos, E. P. (2003). Speech–language pathologists' beliefs about bilingual/bicultural individuals. *American Journal of Speech–Language Pathology, 12,* 73–91.

Kuster, J. M. (2002). Web–based information resources for evidence-based practice in speech–language pathology, *Perspectives on Language Learning and Education, 6,* 6–14

Language Analysis Lab, (2003). *Systematic Analysis of Language Transcripts (SALT) Software.* Retrieved February 19, 2005, from *http://www .languageanalysislab.com/*

LaPointe, L. (1985). Aphasia therapy: Some principles and strategies for treatment. In D. F. Johns (Ed.), *Clinical Management of Neurogenic Communicative Disorders* (pp. 179–241). Boston: Little Brown.

Law, M. (2000). Strategies for implementing evidence-based practice in early intervention. *Infants and Young Children, 13,* 32–40.

Leonard, L. B. (1979). Language impairment in children. *Merrill–Palmer Quarterly, 25,* 205–232.

Leonard, L. B., & Finneran, D. (2003). Grammatical morphemes effects on MLU: "The same can be less" revisited. *Journal of Speech–Language–Hearing Research, 46,* 878–888.

Levin, J. R., & Wampold, B. E. (1999). Generalized single–case randomization tests: Flexible analyses for a variety of situations. *School Psychology Quarterly, 14,* 59–93.

Lincoln, Y. S., & Guba, E. G. (1985). *Naturalistic inquiry.* New York: Sage Publications.

Locke, L., Silverman, S., & Spirduso, W. (1998). *Reading and understanding research.* Thousand Oaks, CA: SAGE Publications.

Locke, L. F. Silverman, S. J., & Spirduso, W. W. (2004). *Reading and understanding research.* Thousand Oaks, CA: Sage Publications.

Logemann, J. A. (1997). Criteria for studies of treatment for oral–pharyngeal dysphagia. *Dysphagia, 1,* 193–199.

Long, S. (2004). *Computerized Profiling.* Retrieved February 19, 2005 from, *http://www. computerizedprofiling.org/*

Lyons, L. C. (2004). *The meta–analysis page.* Retrieved August 26, 2004 from, *http://www. lyonsmorris.com/MetaA/index.htm*

Marvin, L. A., Montano, J. J., Fusco, L. M., & Gould, E. P. (2003). Speech–language pathologists' perceptions of their training and experience in using augmentative and alternative communication. *Contemporary Issues in Communication Science and Disorders, 30,* 76–83.

Mastergeorge, A. M. (1999). Revelations of family perceptions of diagnosis and disorder through metaphor. In D. Kovarsky, J. Duchan, & M. Maxwell (Eds.). Constructing (in)competence: Disabling evaluations in clinical and social interactions (pp. 245–256). Mahwah, NJ: Erlbaum.

Max, L., & Onghena, P. (1999). Some issues in the statistical analysis of completely randomized and repeated measures designs for speech, language, and hearing research. *Journal of Speech–Language–Hearing Research, 42,* 261–270.

McAllister, L. (1998). What constitutes good qualitative research writing—in theses and papers? In Higgs, J. (Ed.) *Writing qualitative research* (pp. 217–232). Sydney, Australia: Hampden Press.

McGregor, K. K., Newman, R. M., Reilly, R. M., & Capone, N. C. (2002). Semantic representation and naming in children with specific language impairment. *Journal of Speech–Language–Hearing Research, 45,* 998–1014.

McGue, M. (2000). Authorship and intellectual property. In B. D. Sales & S. Folkman (Eds.). Ethics in research with human participants (pp. 185–219). Washington, DC: American Psychological Association.

McHenry, M. A. (2003). The effect of pacing strategies on the variability of speech movement sequences in dysarthria. *Journal of Speech–Language–Hearing Research, 46,* 702–710.

Meline, T. (2003). Problems in synthesis (meta–analytic) studies: An example from the communication disorders literature. *Perceptual and Motor Skills, 97,* 1085–1088.

Meline, T., Gonzalez, E., Florez-Sabo, B., & Hinojosa, V. (2004, November). Effects of Paired Reading Practice on Children's Reading Fluency. Poster session presented at the annual meeting of the American Speech-Hearing-Language Association, Philadelphia, PA.

Meline, T., & Mata–Pistokache, T. (2003). The perils of Pauline's e-mail: Professional issues for audiologists and speech–language pathologists. *Contemporary Issues in Communication Science and Disorders, 30,* 118–123.

Meline, T., & Paradiso, T. (2003). Evidence–based practice in schools: Evaluating research and reducing barriers. *Language, Speech, and Hearing Services in Schools, 34,* 273–283.

Meline, T., & Schmitt, J. F. (1997). Case studies for evaluating statistical significance in group designs. *American Journal of Speech–Language Pathology, 6,* 33–41.

Meline, T., & Wang, B. (2004). Effect–size reporting practices in *AJSLP* and other ASHA journals: 1999–2003. *American Journal of Speech–Language Pathology, 13,* 202–207.

Mendes, A. P. (2000). *Informed consent form: Effects of vocal training on respiration, phonation and articulation.* Indiana University of Pennsylvania School of Graduate Studies and Research (model Protocols). Retrieved August 26, 2004 from, *http://www.iup.edu/graduate/irb/models.shtm*

Metz, D. E., & Folkins, J. W. (1985). Protection of human subjects in speech and hearing research. *Asha, 27,* 25–29.

Minitab (1998). *Minitab statistical software release 12.* State College, PA: Minitab Inc.

Mirrett, P. L., Roberts, J. E., & Price, J. (2003). Early intervention practices and communication intervention strategies for young males with Fragile X syndrome. *Language, Speech, and Hearing Services in Schools, 14,* 320–331.

Mizuko, M. & Reichle, J. (1989). Transparency and recall of symbols among intellectually handicapped adults. *Journal of Speech and Hearing Disorders, 54,* 627–633.

Mueller, P. B., & Lisko, D. (2003). Undergraduate research in CSD programs: A solution to the PhD shortage? *Contemporary Issues in Communication Science and Disorders, 30,* 123–126.

Muma, J. (1993). The need for replication. *Journal of Speech and Hearing Research, 36,* 927–930.

Nail-Chiwetalu, B., & Bernstein Ratner, N. (2003). *Fostering information literacy competency.* Proceedings of the Council on Academic Programs in Communication Sciences and Disorders Conference. Retrieved August 26, 2004 from, *http://www.capcsd.org/proceedings/2003/talks/chiwetalu2003.pdf.*

Nathan, L., Stackhouse, J., Goulandris, N., & Snowling, M. J. (2004). The development of early listening skills among children with speech difficulties: A test of the "critical age hypothesis." *Journal of Speech–Language–Hearing Research, 47,* 377–391.

National Institute on Deafness and Other Communication Disorders, (2004). *Guidelines on communicating informed consent for individuals who are deaf or hard–of–hearing and scientists.* Retrieved August 27, 2004 from, *http://www.nidcd.nih.gov/news/releases/99/inform/xviii.asp.*

National Library of Medicine, (2004a). *MeSH.* Retrieved August 26, 2004 from, *http://www.ncbi.nlm.nih.gov.*

National Library of Medicine, (2004b). *National Information Center on Health Services Research and Health Care Technology.* Retrieved August 27, 2004 from, *http://www.nlm.nih.gov/nichsr/nichsr.html.*

National Student Speech Language Hearing Association, (2004). *Publications main page*. Retrieved August 29, 2004 from, *http://www.nsslha.org/NSSLHA/publications*.

NIH Office of Extramural Research, (2000). NIH *guidelines on the inclusion of women and minorities as subjects in clinical research (updated)*. Retrieved August 29, 2004 from, *http://grants.nih.gov/grants/funding/women_min/ guidelines_update.htm*.

Norušis, M. J. (1988). *The SPSS guide to data analysis for SPSS/PC+*. Chicago: SPSS Inc.

Oelschlaeger, M., & Damico, J. S. (2000). Partnership in conversation: A study of word search strategies. *Journal of Communication Disorders, 33*, 205–225.

Office of Behavioral and Social Sciences Research: NIH, (2004). *Qualitative methods in health research: Opportunities and considerations in applications and reviews*. Retrieved August 26, 2004 from, *http://obssr.od.nih.gov/Publications/Qualitative.PDF*.

Office of Human Subjects Research (2004). *Research involving cognitively impaired subjects: A review of some ethical considerations (OHSR information sheet 7)*. Retrieved August 27, 2004 from, *http://www.nihtraining.com/ohsrsite/info/info.html*.

Ohio Board of Speech-Language Pathology and Audiology, (2004). *Ohio Law and Administrative Rules Governing the Practice of Speech-Language Pathology and Audiology*. Retrieved August 27, 2004 from, *http://slpaud.ohio.gov/lawsandrules.htm*.

Olswang, L. B. (1990). Treatment efficacy research: A path to quality assurance. *Asha, 32*, 45–47.

O'Neil-Pirozzi, T. M. (2003). Language Functioning of Residents in Family Homeless Shelters. *American Journal of Speech–Language Pathology, 12*, 229–242.

Orwin, R. G. (1983). A fail-safe *N* for effect size in meta–analysis. *Journal of Educational Statistics, 8*, 157–159.

Paashe-Orlow, M. K., Taylor, H. A., & Brancati, F. L. (2003). Readability standards for informed–consent forms as compared with actual readability. *The New England Journal of Medicine, 348*, 721–726.

Patten, M. L. (2004). *Understanding research methods*. Glendale, CA: Pyrczak Publishing.

Plante, T. G. (1998). Teaching psychology ethics to undergraduates: An experiential model. *Teaching of Psychology, 25*, 281–285.

Preisser, D. A., Hodson, B. W., & Paden, E. P. (1988). Developmental phonology: 18–29 months. *Journal of Speech and Hearing Disorders, 53*, 125–130.

Pyrczak, F., & Bruce, R. R. (2003). *Writing empirical research reports*. Los Angeles: Pyrczak Publishing.

Qualitative Interest Group, (2004). *Purpose, history and activities*. Retrieved August 26, 2004, from University of Georgia College of Education Web Site: *http://www.coe.uga.edu/quig/archives/index.html*

Reid, R., Hertzog, M., & Snyder, M. (1996). Educating every teacher, every year: The public schools and parents of children with ADHD. *Seminars in Speech and Language, 17*, 73–87.

Reilly, S., Douglas, J., & Oates, J. (2004). *Evidence based practice in speech pathology*. Philadelphia: Whurr Publishers.

Reynolds, M. E., Callihan, K., & Browning, E. (2003). Effect of instruction on the development of rhyming skills in young children. *Contemporary Issues in Communication Science and Disorders, 30*, 41–46.

Robey, R. R. (1998). A meta–analysis of clinical outcomes in the treatment of aphasia. *Journal of Speech–Language–Hearing Research, 41*, 172–187.

Robey, R. R., & Dalebout, S. D. (1998). A tutorial on conducting meta–analysis of clinical outcome research. *Journal of Speech–Language–Hearing Research, 41*, 1227–1241.

Robey, R. R., & Schultz, M. C. (1998). A model for conducting clinical–outcome research: An adaptation of the standard protocol for use in aphasiology. *Aphasiology, 12*, 787–810.

Robey, R. R., Schultz, M. C., Crawford, A. B., & Sinner, C. A. (1999). Single–subject clinical–outcome research: Designs, data, effect sizes, and analyses. *Aphasiology, 13*, 445–473.

Rodriguez, B. L., & Olswang, L. B. (2003). Mexican–American and Anglo–American mothers' beliefs and values about child rearing, education, and language impairment. *American Journal of Speech–Language Pathology, 12*, 452–462.

Rosenberg, M. S., Adams, D. C., & Gurevitch, J. (2000). *MetaWin: Statistical software for meta–analysis version 2.0.* Sunderland, MA: Sinauer Associates.

Roy, N., Weinrich, B., Gray, S. D., Tanner, K., Stemple, J. C., & Sapienza, C. M. (2003). Three treatments for teachers with voice disorders: A randomized clinical trial. *Journal of Speech–Language–Hearing Research, 46*, 670–688.

Sapir, S., Spielman, J., Ramig, L. O., Hinds, S., Countryman, S., Fox, C., Story, B. (2003). Effects of intensive voice treatment (the Lee Silverman Voice Treatment [LSVT]) on ataxic dysarthria: A case study. *American Journal of Speech–Language Pathology, 12*, 387–399.

Schlosser, R. W., & Blischak, D. M. (2004). Effects of speech and print feedback on spelling by children with autism. *Journal of Speech–Language–Hearing Research, 47*, 848–862.

Schmitt, J. F., & Meline, T. J. (1990). Subject descriptions, control groups, and research designs in published studies of language–impaired children. *Journal of Communication Disorders, 23*, 365–382.

Scruggs, T. E., & Mastropieri, M. A. (2001). How to summarize single–participant research: Ideas and applications. *Exceptionality, 9*, 227–244.

Shadish, W. R., Cook, T. D., & Campbell, D. T. (2002). *Experimental and quasi–experimental designs for generalized causal inference.* Boston: Houghton–Mifflin.

Shalala, D. (2000). Protecting research subjects— What must be done. *New England Journal of Medicine, 343*, 808–810.

Shriberg, L. D., & Kwiatkowski, J. (1987). A retrospective study of spontaneous generalization in speech–delayed children. *Language, Speech, and Hearing Services in Schools, 18*, 144–157.

Simmons-Mackie, N. N., & Damico, J. S. (2003). Contributions of qualitative research to the knowledge base of normal communication. *American Journal of Speech–Language Pathology, 12*, 144–154.

Sininger, Y., Marsh, R., Walden, B., & Wilber, L. A. (2003). Guidelines for ethical practice in research for audiologists. *Audiology Today, 15*, 14–17.

Smith, G. D., Egger, M., & Phillips, A. N. (1997). Meta–analysis: Beyond the grand mean? *BMJ, 315*, 1600–1614.

Smith-Olinde, L., Besing, J., & Koehnke, J. (2004). Interference and enhancement effects on interaural time discrimination and level discrimination in listeners with normal hearing and those with hearing loss. *American Journal of Speech–Language Pathology, 13*, 80–95.

Southwood, F., & Russell, A. F. (2004). Comparison of conversation, freeplay, and story generation as methods of language sample elicitation. *Journal of Speech–Language–Hearing Research, 47*, 366–376.

State of Illinois Division of Professional Regulations, (2004). *Section 1465.95 Professional Conduct Standards.* Retrieved August 26, 2004 from, *http://www.ildpr.com/WHO/ar/spchpath.asp.*

Sternberg, R. J. (1992). How to win acceptance by psychology journals: Twenty–one tips for better writing. *APS Observer, 12*, 13, 18.

Sternberg, R. J. (1993). *The psychologist's companion: A guide to scientific writing for students and researchers.* New York: Cambridge University Press.

Stewart, M., Pankiw, R., Lehman, M. E., & Simpson, T. H. (2002). Hearing loss and hearing handicap in users of recreational firearms. *Journal of the American Academy of Audiology, 13*, 160–168.

Stillman, R., Snow, R., & Warren, K. (1999). "I used to be good with kids." Encounters between speech–language pathology students and children with pervasive developmental disorders (PDD). In D. Kovarsky, J. Duchan, & M. Maxwell (Eds.). *Constructing (in)competence: Disabling evaluations in clinical and social interaction* (pp. 29–48). Mahwah, NJ: Erlbaum.

Strum, J. M., & Nelson, N. W. (1997). Formal classroom lessons: New perspectives on a familiar discourse event. *Language, Speech, and Hearing Services in Schools, 28,* 255–273.

Stuart, A. (2004). An investigation of list equivalency of the Northwestern University Auditory Test No. 6 in interrupted broadband noise. *American Journal of Audiology, 13,* 23–28.

Tetnowski, J. A., & Franklin, T. C. (2003). Qualitative research: Implications for description and assessment. *American Journal of Speech–Language Pathology, 12,* 155–164.

Tharpe, A. M., & Ashmead, D. H. (2001). A longitudinal investigation of infant auditory sensitivity. *American Journal of Audiology, 10,* 1–9.

Todman, J. B., & Dugard, P. (2001). Single–case and small–n experimental designs: A practical guide to randomization tests. Mahwah, NJ: Lawrence Erlbaum.

Trochim, B. (2004). *Bill Trochim's center for social research methods.* Retrieved August 26, 2004 from, *http://trochim.human.cornell.edu*

Turkstra, L., Ciccia, A., & Seaton, C. (2003). Interactive behaviors in adolescent conversation dyads. *Language, Speech, and Hearing Services in Schools, 34,* 117–127.

Tyler, A. A., Lewis, K. E., Haskill, A., & Tolbert, L. C. (2003). Outcomes of different speech and language goal attack strategies. *Journal of Speech–Language–Hearing Research, 46,* 1077–1094.

Ukrainetz, T. A., & Fresquez, E. F. (2003). "What *isn't* language?": A qualitative study of the role of the school speech–language pathologist. *Language, Speech, and Hearing Services in Schools, 34,* 284–298.

U. S. Department of Health and Human Services, (1990, September 28). ADAMHA/NIH policy concerning inclusion of minorities in study populations. *NIH Guide for Grants and Contracts, 19,* 1–2.

Waddell, C. (2004). *Thesis writing.* Retrieved November 26, 2004 from, *http://www.rpi.edu/web/writingcenter/thesis.html*

Wadsworth, B. J. (1989). *Piaget's theory of cognitive and affective development.* New York: Longman.

Walden, B. E., Surr, R. K., Cord, M. T., & Dyrlund, O. (2004). Predicting hearing aid microphone preference in everyday listening. *Journal of the American Academy of Audiology, 15,* 365–396.

Walden, T. C., & Walden, B. E. (2004). Predicting success with hearing aids in everyday living. *Journal of the American Academy of Audiology, 15,* 342–352.

Walters, D. B., & Chapman, R. S. (2000). Comprehension monitoring: A developmental effect? *American Journal of Speech–Language Pathology, 9,* 48–54.

Walton, J. H., McCardle, P., Crowe, T. A., & Wilson, B. E. (1990). Black English in a Mississippi prison population. *Journal of Speech and Hearing Disorders, 55,* 206–216.

Wambaugh, J., & Bain, B. (2002). Make research methods an integral part of your clinical practice. *ASHA Leader Online.* Retrieved August 26, 2004 from, *http://www.asha.org/about/publications/leader-online/archives/2002/q4/021119.htm.*

Weaver-Spurlock, S., & Brasseur, J. (1988). The effects of simultaneous sound–position training on the generalization of [s]. *Language, Speech, and Hearing Services in Schools, 19,* 259–271.

Wertz, R. T., LaPointe, L. L., & Rosenbeck, J. C. (1984). Apraxia of speech in adults: The disorder and its management. Needham Heights, MA: Allyn and Bacon.

White House OPS (Office of the Press Secretary), (1997, May 16). *Remarks by the President in apology for study done in Tuskegee.* Retrieved August 26, 2004 from, *http://clinton4.nara.gov/textonly/New/Remarks/Fri/19970516 -898.html.*

Williams, A. L. (2000). Multiple oppositions: Case studies of variables in phonological interven-

tion. *American Journal of Speech–Language Pathology, 9,* 289–299.

Williams, A. L., & Elbert, M. (2003). A prospective longitudinal study of phonological development in late talkers. *Language, Speech, and Hearing Services in Schools, 34,* 138–153.

Williams, A. L., & Fagelson, M. (2003). Fostering a community of scholars in a graduate program. *ASHA Leader Online.* Retrieved August 26, 2004 from, *http://www.asha.org/about/publications/leader-online/archives/2003/q1/030304fa.htm*

Yairi, E., Watkins, R., Ambrose, N., & Paden, E. (2001). What is stuttering? *Journal of Speech–Language–Hearing Research, 44,* 585–592.

Yoder, P. J. (1989). Maternal question use predicts later language development in specific–language–disordered children. *Journal of Speech and Hearing Disorders, 54,* 347–355.

Yorkston, K. M., Smith, K., & Beukelman, D. (1990). Extended communication samples of augmented communicators I: A comparison of individualized versus standard single–word vocabularies. *Journal of Speech and Hearing Disorders, 55,* 217–224.

AUTHOR INDEX

SUBJECT INDEX